GENTLE WALL PILATES FOR SENIORS:

BUILDING CORE STRENGTH, BALANCE, FLEXIBILITY, IMPROVE SLEEP QUALITY AND ENHANCED EMOTIONAL WELL-BEING FOR A HEALTHIER AGING PROCESS

EVA STRONG

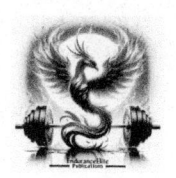

© COPYRIGHT EVA STRONG 2024
- ALL RIGHTS RESERVED

The content within this book may not be reproduced, duplicated, or transmitted without direct written permission from the author or the publisher.

Under no circumstances will any blame or legal responsibility be held against the publisher or author for any damages, reparation, or monetary loss due to the information contained within this book. Either directly or indirectly. You are responsible for your own choices, actions, and results.

Legal Notice:

This book is copyright-protected. This book is only for personal use. You cannot amend, distribute, sell, use, quote, or paraphrase any part of this book's content without the author's or publisher's consent.

Disclaimer Notice:

Please note the information contained within this document is for educational and entertainment purposes only. All effort has been expended to present accurate, up-to-date, reliable, and complete information. No warranties of any kind are declared or implied. Readers acknowledge that the author is not engaging in rendering legal, financial, medical, or professional advice. The content within this book has been derived from various sources. Please consult a licensed professional before attempting any techniques outlined in this book.

By reading this document, the reader agrees that under no circumstances is the author responsible for any losses, direct or indirect, which are incurred as a result of the use of the information contained within this document, including, but not limited to, — errors, omissions, or inaccuracies.

CONTENTS

Introduction	vii
1. FOUNDATIONAL KNOWLEDGE	1
1.1 Pilates: A Historical Perspective Tailored for Seniors	1
1.2 The Science of Aging and Pilates' Role in Longevity	3
1.3 Decoding the Principles of Pilates for the Senior Body	6
1.4 Overcoming the Myth: "Too Old for Pilates"	8
1.5 The Interplay of Mind and Body in Senior Pilates Practice	11
1.6 Understanding Your Body's Needs and Pilates' Solutions	13
1.7 The Benefits of Pilates on Mental Health for Seniors	15
1.8 Safety First: Preventing Injury with Proper Technique	17
1.9 Adapting Pilates for Various Senior Fitness Levels	20
1.10 Pilates and Chronic Conditions: A Gentle Approach	22
2. GENTLE WALL PILATES FOR SENIORS: BUILDING STRENGTH AND STABILITY	25
2.1 Basic Wall Exercises	26
2.2 Building Core Strength Without the Floor: Wall-Based Exercises	28
2.3 Enhancing Flexibility and Range of Motion Gently	31
2.4 Balance and Stability Through Wall Pilates	35
2.5 Breathwork and Pilates: Enhancing Lung Capacity and Relaxation	38
2.6 Tailoring Pilates to Address Lower Back Pain	41
2.7 Pilates Movements for Improving Posture in Seniors	44
2.8 The Role of Pilates in Managing Arthritis Pain	47
2.9 Pilates for Osteoporosis: Safe Practices for Bone Health	50
2.10 Mobility and Independence: Pilates Exercises That Empower	55
3. DESIGNING A PERSONAL PILATES AREA AT HOME	59
3.1 Incorporating Pilates into Your Daily Routine	63
3.2 Short and Sweet: The 10-Minute Pilates Workout for Busy Days	65
3.3 From Morning to Night: Pilates Throughout the Day	67

3.4 Engaging with Technology: Using Apps for Progress Tracking	70
3.5 The Power of Habit: Making Pilates a Daily Ritual	72
3.6 Pilates and Socialization: Forming Your Support Group	74
3.7 Staying Motivated: Celebrating Milestones and Progress	76
3.8 Adapting Your Pilates Practice as You Age	78
3.9 Pilates for the Mind: Combining Meditation and Movement	80
4. DIVERSIFYING YOUR PILATES TOOLKIT	**86**
Am I Ready for Pilates Equipment?	88
4.1 Chair Pilates: An Accessible Alternative for Enhanced Mobility	92
4.2 Combining Pilates with Other Low-Impact Exercises	97
4.3 Advanced Stretching Techniques for Flexibility	103
4.4 The Role of Resistance Bands in Pilates Progression	105
4.5 Pilates Sequences for Every Season of the Year	108
4.6 Overcoming Plateaus: Tips for Continued Improvement	110
4.7 Pilates for Balance and Coordination: Advanced Techniques	112
4.8 The Future of Pilates in Senior Fitness: Trends and Innovations	115
4.9 Pilates Retreats and Workshops: Deepening Your Practice	117
5. EMBRACING A PILATES LIFESTYLE: NOURISHING BODY AND MIND	**120**
5.1 The Impact of Pilates on Sleep and Relaxation	125
5.2 Building a Community Through Pilates	127
5.3 Pilates as a Catalyst for Lifestyle Change	129
5.4 The Legacy of Pilates in Senior Wellness: Looking Forward	131
6. BEGINNERS WALL PILATES 10-MINUTE ROUTINE	**133**
Day 1: Introduction to Wall Pilates	134
Day 2: Core and Legs	137
Day 3: Flexibility and Balance	139
Day 4: Upper Body and Posture	141
Day 5: Core Engagement and Stability	144
Day 6: Balance and Coordination	146
Day 7: Gentle Stretch and Relaxation	149

Conclusion	153
Frequently Asked Questions	155
Fitness Tracker and Monthly Calendar	163
References	167

INTRODUCTION

Let me share a story that perfectly captures what we'll dive into. It's about Joan, a vibrant 72-year-old who thought her days of feeling solid and flexible were well behind her. After discovering Pilates, Joan experienced a transformation that wasn't just physical - it was a profound reclaiming of her vitality and zest for life. Through Pilates, she regained flexibility and strength and found a new sense of balance and inner peace that she thought was lost to age. This story isn't just about Joan; it's a testament to the transformative power of Pilates for seniors, and it's exactly the journey I want to guide you through in this book.

I fervently believe in the power of movement and fitness at any age, with a passion for empowering seniors through Pilates. My mission, aligned with EndureElite Publications, is to provide accessible, high-quality fitness guides that make a real difference in your life. This book embodies our shared mission, designed to introduce you, our senior readers, to the wonders of Pilates, ensuring that each exercise is achievable and enjoyable, regardless of your current fitness level.

Our primary goal with this book is straightforward: to provide you with a comprehensive guide to practicing Pilates, specifically tailored for the aging body. We're focusing on low-impact, accessible exercises catering to various fitness levels, from beginners to more advanced. It's

INTRODUCTION

all about creating a safer, healthier, and more vibrant aging process for you.

To all the seniors out there, I know the unique challenges and aspirations you face when staying active. Starting your Pilates journey is always possible. Through this book, you'll discover structured exercise routines explained in a way that's easy to understand and diverse enough to keep you engaged and looking forward to your next workout.

What sets this book apart is its unique features, like combining Pilates with other exercises to keep your workouts fresh and effective, no matter how much time you have on your hands. Expect short, impactful workouts with progress-tracking tools to support your physical and mental well-being.

My philosophy on fitness and aging is simple: it's a lifelong adventure, not a fleeting pursuit. Sustainable fitness practices and celebrating every milestone are at the core of this journey. This philosophy permeates every page of this book, encouraging you to embrace each step of your Pilates path with joy and determination.

As for the book's structure, it's designed to be your roadmap through the world of Pilates for seniors, covering everything from the basics to more advanced techniques, all while keeping your unique needs in mind.

And before we embark on this journey together, let me share a personal anecdote. My introduction to Pilates came later in life, and it was a humbling experience. I realized that age is just a number. Each Pilates session made me feel more robust, flexible, and, most importantly, more connected to my body. This personal journey has inspired me to share the gift of Pilates with you.

Renowned Pilates expert Joseph Pilates once said, "Physical fitness is the first requisite of happiness." This quote perfectly encapsulates the heart of Pilates for seniors. It's adaptable, it's empowering, and it has the potential to enhance your health and well-being significantly.

So, with an open mind and a willing heart, I invite you to join me on this Pilates journey. Together, we'll explore how Pilates can transform your body and enrich your life, proving that the best years are not behind us but are happening now. Let's get started.

1

FOUNDATIONAL KNOWLEDGE

In fitness and well-being, certain truths are universal, transcending age, time, and geographical boundaries. Among these, the quest for exercise that nurtures both body and mind without the harsh impact of more vigorous activities stands out, especially for those in their golden years. This search leads many to the doorstep of Pilates, a method not just born out of necessity but thrived on the principle of thoughtful, deliberate movement. With its unique blend of strength, flexibility, and mindfulness, Pilates has woven its way into the fabric of fitness regimes worldwide, becoming particularly cherished among seniors. The beauty of Pilates lies not only in its historical richness but in its adaptability, making it a perfect fit for those seeking gentle yet effective ways to stay active.

1.1 PILATES: A HISTORICAL PERSPECTIVE TAILORED FOR SENIORS

Historical Evolution

The inception of Pilates, dating back to the early 20th century, was the brainchild of Joseph Pilates, a man ahead of his time who believed in the power of the mind to control the muscles. His method, termed initially "Contrology," was a response to the physical and mental ailments he observed around him, compounded by his experiences with illness and physical weaknesses in his youth. Pilates developed his method as a form of exercise and a comprehensive physical and mental conditioning system. This system emphasizes controlled movements and breathing to strengthen the body's core, improve posture, and promote efficient, graceful movement.

Joseph Pilates' Vision

Joseph Pilates envisioned a workout routine that transcended age barriers and could be modified and adapted to cater to anyone, including seniors. His vision was deeply personal, rooted in his journey to transform physical health through disciplined exercise and mindfulness. Pilates believed in the interconnectivity of physical and mental health, advocating for a balanced approach to well-being that considered the whole person. His revolutionary methodology offered a gentle yet challenging way to maintain strength, flexibility, and vitality.

Adapting to Modern Needs

As Pilates' methodology traversed through time, it evolved, adapting to the changing needs of society and the growing body of scientific knowledge about health and fitness. Today, Pilates encompasses a spectrum of exercises that can be performed on a mat or specialized equipment, such as the reformer, which adds resistance to the exercises. This adaptability makes Pilates appealing to seniors, who often recommend low-impact exercises. Modern Pilates instructors are trained to modify exercises to accommodate individual needs, including seniors with chronic conditions or mobility issues. This bespoke approach ensures that Pilates remains inclusive, safe, and beneficial for aging bodies, aligning perfectly with contemporary understandings of senior health and fitness.

The Growth in Popularity Among Seniors

The surge in Pilates' popularity among the senior demographic is not coincidental but a testament to its relevance and effectiveness. Seniors find Pilates a pathway to maintaining agility, improving balance, and enhancing overall well-being without the risk of injury associated with high-impact exercises. Pilates offers more than just physical benefits; it also provides a mental workout, encouraging practitioners to focus on their breathing and the precise execution of movements. This mindfulness aspect helps reduce stress and promote a sense of calm, contributing to a holistic approach to aging well.

One significant factor contributing to Pilates' appeal is its emphasis on core strength. A strong core is crucial for maintaining balance and preventing falls, a common concern for many seniors. Moreover, the controlled, flowing movements in Pilates help improve joint mobility and flexibility, which can be particularly beneficial for those with arthritis or stiffness. The breathing techniques taught in Pilates also play a vital role in enhancing lung capacity and circulation, which are essential for overall health and vitality.

Pilates' adaptability means that it can be practiced almost anywhere, from the comfort of one's home to specialized studios and even outdoors. This flexibility, combined with the minimal equipment required for mat exercises, makes Pilates an accessible option for seniors looking to integrate regular physical activity into their lives. Furthermore, the Pilates community, with its supportive instructors and fellow practitioners, offers a sense of belonging and motivation, enriching the experience beyond the physical exercises.

As we delve deeper into the following chapters, we'll explore the specific Pilates exercises most beneficial for seniors, the science behind the method, and practical tips for incorporating Pilates into everyday life. The journey through Pilates is one of discovery and transformation, offering a path to a healthier, more vibrant aging process grounded in the wisdom of its founder and tailored to the needs of today's seniors.

1.2 THE SCIENCE OF AGING AND PILATES' ROLE IN LONGEVITY

Aging naturally brings about a series of changes in both physical and mental health. These changes can often lead to decreased activity levels, but it doesn't have to be an inevitable decline. Pilates, with its focus on controlled movements and core strength, plays a pivotal role in navigating the aging process more smoothly, offering a way to mitigate some common health issues associated with aging.

Biological Impacts of Aging

As individuals age, they often experience a decline in muscle mass and bone density, leading to decreased mobility and an increased risk of fractures. The body's metabolism also slows down, contributing to weight gain and associated health issues like diabetes and heart disease. On the mental front, cognitive functions can decline, and there are increased risks of depression and loneliness due to lifestyle changes like retirement or the loss of loved ones.

Pilates addresses these physical changes by promoting muscle strength and flexibility, which can help counteract the loss of muscle mass and bone density. The emphasis on core strength aids in improving posture and balance, reducing the risk of falls—a common concern for many seniors. Moreover, the focused nature of Pilates exercises encourages mindfulness. It can positively impact mental well-being, helping to keep the mind sharp and alleviate feelings of depression.

Pilates for Enhanced Mobility and Strength

Focusing on the core, Pilates exercises are uniquely designed to build strength in the muscles surrounding the spine, hips, and shoulders, areas crucial for maintaining mobility and balance. The exercises are often performed in a flowing sequence that mimics daily movements, improving functional fitness and making everyday tasks more accessible and safer.

Pilates also emphasizes slow, controlled movements that increase muscular strength without the strain of high-impact exercises. This gentle approach makes it ideal for seniors who may be dealing with joint pain or osteoarthritis. Pilates helps seniors maintain their independence by improving muscle strength and flexibility, contributing to a higher quality of life.

Preventive Benefits

Regular Pilates practice offers several preventive benefits for common age-related issues:

•**Falls and Loss of Balance:** Pilates improves balance and coordination, significantly reducing the risk of falls. Exercises focusing on the core and legs strengthen the body's stabilizing muscles, making it easier to maintain balance during movement and while stationary.

•**Osteoporosis:** Weight-bearing and resistance exercises in Pilates stimulate bone growth, helping to prevent bone density loss. While traditional Pilates practices include many non-weight-bearing exercises, modifications, and equipment like the Pilates Reformer can incorporate the necessary resistance to aid bone health.

•**Joint Health:** Pilates promotes a full range of motion in the joints, which is crucial for keeping joints healthy and fluid. The controlled movements help lubricate joint areas, reducing the risk of stiffness and pain associated with arthritis.

Supporting Longevity and Quality of Life

Numerous studies point to the effectiveness of Pilates in supporting a longer, healthier life. Research has shown that regular Pilates practice can significantly improve balance, flexibility, and muscle strength among older adults. These factors directly contribute to longevity and the prevention of injuries. Furthermore, Pilates has been linked to improved cardiovascular health, a key component of longevity.

One study found that participants improved lower body strength, flexibility, and balance after practicing Pilates regularly, decreasing fall risk. Another important aspect of Pilates is its ability to be adapted to each individual's fitness level and health conditions, ensuring that everyone, regardless of their starting point, can benefit from the practice.

Pilates supports physical health and significantly affects mental and emotional well-being. The focus on breathing and mindfulness during Pilates sessions helps to reduce stress and anxiety, which are common as people age. This mental clarity and relaxation can lead to better sleep patterns and overall well-being, contributing to a happier, more fulfilled life.

By engaging in Pilates, seniors can actively participate in their health and well-being, combating the natural effects of aging with grace and strength. Pilates offers a comprehensive approach to aging, whether maintaining muscle mass and flexibility, improving balance to prevent falls, or simply enjoying the mental clarity from a focused workout. Its adaptability makes it a sustainable practice for life, continuously supporting seniors in their quest for longevity and quality of life. Through regular Pilates practice, aging can transform from a series of challenges to an opportunity for growth, empowerment, and well-being.

1.3 DECODING THE PRINCIPLES OF PILATES FOR THE SENIOR BODY

Pilates stands out as a form of exercise that equally engages the mind and the body, anchored in principles that foster a deep connection between the two. For seniors especially, understanding and applying these principles can significantly enhance the effectiveness and benefits of their Pilates practice. Let's explore how these foundational elements of Pilates cater to the aging body and contribute to a holistic fitness approach.

Core Principles of Pilates

At the heart of Pilates are six principles that guide every movement, ensuring that the practice is more than just physical exercise—it becomes a form of moving meditation that nurtures both the body and the mind.

- **Centering:** This principle focuses on the 'powerhouse' of the body—the center, encompassing the abdomen, lower back, hips, and buttocks. For seniors, centering is crucial for improving core strength, which is essential for balance and stability, reducing the risk of falls.
- **Concentration:** Pilates demands focused attention on each movement, engaging the mind with the body. This concentration enhances body awareness, allowing seniors to perform exercises with better form and reduced risk of injury.
- **Control:** Every Pilates exercise is performed with complete muscular control, eliminating careless, hasty movements. Control is particularly beneficial for seniors, ensuring movements are safe and effective, tailored to their strength and flexibility levels.
- **Precision:** Precision in Pilates means executing each movement with intention and exactness. This principle helps the senior population fine-tune motor skills, improve coordination, and maintain joint health.

- **Breath:** Breathing in Pilates is not an afterthought but a vital component of the exercises. Proper breathing techniques enhance oxygen circulation and support the core muscles, aiding seniors in executing movements more efficiently.
- **Flow:** The principle of flow refers to the smooth transition between exercises, creating a sequence that feels like a continuous movement. Flow keeps the heart rate up and promotes endurance, vital for seniors' cardiovascular health.

Adaptation to Senior Needs

Adapting these principles to meet the needs of seniors ensures that Pilates remains an accessible and beneficial practice for this age group. Here are some modifications that can be made:

- **Modified Centering:** For seniors, particularly those with back issues, centering exercises can be modified to be performed in a seated or standing position, reducing strain on the back while strengthening the core.
- **Focused Concentration with Visuals:** Utilizing visuals or guided imagery can help seniors maintain concentration, which is especially useful for those who might find maintaining focus challenging.
- **Controlled Movements with Props:** Using props like balls or bands can aid seniors in maintaining control over their movements, providing additional support and resistance.
- **Precision with Props:** Props can also assist in achieving precision in movements, guiding seniors' limbs into the correct alignment and helping them understand the spatial orientation of their bodies.
- **Adapted Breathing:** Breathing exercises might need to be adapted for seniors with respiratory conditions, focusing on gentle, shallow breaths that still support the movement.
- **Flow with Pauses:** Incorporating brief pauses between exercises can help seniors maintain the flow without fatigue, ensuring they can complete the sequence without strain.

Holistic Approach to Senior Fitness

The holistic nature of Pilates, rooted in its principles, makes it an ideal exercise regime for seniors. It's not just about physical fitness; it's about cultivating a mindset that values and integrates the health of the mind and the body. This approach resonates with seniors, who often seek forms of exercise that offer more than just physical benefits. Pilates, emphasizing mindful movement, breathwork, and mental focus, provides a comprehensive fitness solution that addresses the multifaceted aspects of aging, including mental agility, emotional well-being, and social engagement.

Building a Foundation

For seniors embarking on their Pilates journey, grasping these core principles is the first step toward a safe and effective practice. Understanding the 'why' behind each movement enriches the Pilates experience, transforming it from a series of exercises into a meaningful practice that supports overall well-being. Seniors must approach Pilates patiently, allowing themselves the time to learn and internalize these principles. This foundation ensures their safety during the practice. It maximizes the benefits of Pilates, making it a sustainable part of their fitness regimen.

As seniors integrate these principles into their Pilates practice, they'll discover a form of exercise that adapts to their unique bodies and needs, offering a path to improved health, enhanced mobility, and a more profound sense of well-being. The adaptation of Pilates for seniors is not about simplification but about customization, ensuring that every movement and every breath brings them closer to their fitness and wellness goals. This tailored approach, grounded in the holistic principles of Pilates, empowers seniors to maintain their independence, enjoy a vibrant quality of life, and meet the challenges of aging with strength, grace, and resilience.

1.4 OVERCOMING THE MYTH: "TOO OLD FOR PILATES"

The belief that Pilates—or any form of exercise, for that matter—is only for the young and already fit is a myth that needs to be dispelled. It's a narrative that not only discourages many seniors from exploring the benefits of Pilates but also overlooks the adaptability and inclusiveness at the core of this practice. Let's set the record straight and affirm that age should never hinder improving one's health and well-being through Pilates.

Dispelling Age-Related Myths

It's common to hear concerns about being "too old" to start a new physical activity, suggesting a misunderstanding of what Pilates truly represents. Pilates, fundamentally, is about creating a harmonious connection between mind and body through controlled, mindful movements. This principle applies universally, irrespective of age. The adaptability of Pilates means it can be tailored to the unique needs and limitations of an older body, focusing on improving mobility, flexibility, and strength in a gentle yet effective way.

Many might need more strength and flexibility. However, Pilates is not about performing perfect movements from the get-go but about gradual improvement and personal growth. Focusing on core strength, balance, and posture is particularly beneficial for seniors, addressing common age-related issues such as lower back pain and balance difficulties.

Success Stories

Real-life examples are powerful motivation and evidence that starting Pilates later in life can lead to significant health benefits. Consider the story of a community group of seniors who took up Pilates as a way to stay active and social. Within months, members reported physical improvements like better balance, reduced joint pain, and mental health benefits such as decreased stress and a stronger sense of community.

Another notable example is a senior who turned to Pilates after a fall that resulted in a fear of injury. Through gentle, personalized Pilates exercises, they regained confidence in their mobility, significantly reducing the risk of future falls and reclaiming their independence.

The Role of Instructors

The importance of finding a qualified instructor who understands the nuances of teaching Pilates to seniors cannot be overstated. A knowledgeable instructor will ensure that exercises are performed safely and be adept at modifying to accommodate individual needs and limitations. This personalized approach is critical to making Pilates accessible and enjoyable for seniors, helping them gain the most from their practice.

When searching for an instructor, seniors should seek someone with specific experience or training in working with older adults. It's also important to communicate openly with your instructor about any health issues or concerns so they can tailor the sessions accordingly. A good instructor will foster a supportive environment where seniors feel empowered to progress at their own pace.

Starting Your Journey at Any Age

For seniors interested in starting Pilates, here are some practical steps to begin:

- **Research Local Studios and Classes:** Look for Pilates studios or community centers that offer classes specifically designed for seniors. These classes are more likely to move at a pace that's comfortable for beginners and will be more tailored to the needs of older adults.
- **Consider Private Sessions:** If you're particularly concerned about health issues or want a program customized to your needs, private sessions with a certified Pilates instructor might be a good starting point.
- **Start Slowly:** Begin with basic exercises and focus on learning the correct form. Pilates is about more than how much you can do but doing what you can with precision and control.
- **Listen to Your Body:** Always pay attention to how your body feels during and after exercises. Pilates should not cause pain. If something hurts, speak up so your instructor can modify the exercise.
- **Be Consistent:** Consistency is critical to seeing progress in Pilates. Try incorporating Pilates into your routine several times a week, even if it's just a few minutes each day.
- **Stay Positive:** Remember that progress in Pilates, as with anything new, takes time and patience. Celebrate the small victories along the way, whether noticing improved posture, greater flexibility, or simply feeling more connected to your body.

Starting Pilates as a senior is about enhancing physical health and a journey towards a more mindful, balanced lifestyle. With the proper guidance, modifications, and mindset, Pilates can be a rewarding addition to a senior's routine, offering a way to age gracefully, actively, and healthily. The stories of those who have found joy and strength in Pilates later in life testify that it's never too late to start.

1.5 THE INTERPLAY OF MIND AND BODY IN SENIOR PILATES PRACTICE

The fusion of mental and physical exercise in Pilates offers a unique advantage, especially for seniors. This symbiotic relationship between mind and body forms the cornerstone of Pilates, making it more than just a physical workout. It becomes a holistic practice that nourishes the mind as much as it strengthens the body.

Mind-Body Connection

The concept of the mind-body connection has been introduced previously, but Pilates brings it into sharp focus. Each movement in Pilates requires attention and precision, fostering an acute awareness of the body's movements and alignment. This heightened body awareness can translate into better balance and coordination for seniors, reducing the risk of falls and injuries. More so, this connection encourages mental training akin to meditation, where focusing on breath and movement can clear the mind, reduce stress, and elevate mood.

Mental Health Benefits

The benefits of Pilates extend far beyond physical fitness, particularly impacting mental health positively. For seniors, the mental health benefits are manifold:

- **Stress Reduction:** The emphasis on controlled breathing and focused movement helps calm the mind, reducing stress levels. This calming effect can be particularly beneficial for seniors dealing with the day-to-day stresses of aging, health concerns, and lifestyle changes.
- **Improved Focus:** Pilates requires concentration and precision, which can help sharpen focus and attention. Over time, this enhanced focus can spill over into daily activities, making tasks easier and more enjoyable.
- **Decreased Symptoms of Depression and Anxiety:** Regular Pilates practice can lead to significant reductions in symptoms of depression and anxiety. Combining physical activity, focused breathing, and the calming environment often associated with Pilates classes contributes to overall well-being.

Cognitive Function

Research into the impact of Pilates on cognitive function has yielded promising results. Studies suggest regular Pilates practice can enhance seniors' memory, executive function, and cognitive flexibility. This might be attributed to several factors inherent in Pilates practice:

- **Increased Blood Flow:** The physical activity involved in Pilates boosts blood flow to the brain, which can enhance cognitive function.
- **Neuroplasticity:** Engaging in a new physical activity like Pilates can stimulate the brain, promoting neuroplasticity, which is the brain's ability to form new neural connections. This process is essential for learning new skills and maintaining cognitive health.
- **Stress Reduction:** The stress-reducing aspects of Pilates can also play a role in cognitive health. Chronic stress has been linked to cognitive decline, so activities that reduce stress can protect brain health.

Incorporating Mindfulness

Mindfulness in Pilates goes beyond mere concentration on movements. It involves being fully present in the moment, aware of each breath, and attuned to the sensations in the body. Incorporating mindfulness into Pilates practice can deepen the mind-body connection, enhancing the mental and physical benefits of the exercises. Here are some ways seniors can integrate mindfulness into their Pilates routine:

- **Start with Intention:** Begin each Pilates session by setting an intention. This could be as simple as focusing on your breath throughout the practice or being kind to your body by not pushing too hard.
- **Focus on Breath:** Pay close attention to your breathing, not just as a component of the exercises but as a practice in mindfulness. Notice the rhythm of your breath, how it feels as it moves in and out of your body, and how it helps you move more deeply into each exercise.
- **Be Present:** During Pilates practice, keep your mind from wandering to the past or future. When you notice your thoughts drifting, gently bring your focus back to your breath and the movement you're performing.
- **Reflect Post-Practice:** Reflect on your practice for a few moments after your Pilates session. Notice how your body feels, acknowledge any emotions that arise, and appreciate the effort you've put into your practice.

Incorporating these mindfulness practices into Pilates can make each session a meditative experience, offering seniors a powerful tool for enhancing physical health while promoting mental clarity and emotional calmness. This holistic approach to fitness sets Pilates apart, making it an ideal practice for those seeking a balanced and mindful approach to aging. Through Pilates, seniors can cultivate a deep connection to their bodies, empowering them to move through their golden years with strength, grace, and tranquility.

1.6 UNDERSTANDING YOUR BODY'S NEEDS AND PILATES' SOLUTIONS

Embarking on a Pilates program explicitly crafted for seniors starts with recognizing that each individual brings a unique set of physical conditions, capabilities, and health concerns to the mat. This diversity demands a tailored approach to exercise, ensuring that every senior can experience the full benefits of Pilates without risk of discomfort or injury.

Individual Physical Assessment

Before diving into Pilates, taking stock of one's physical health through an assessment is crucial. This could involve a check-up with a healthcare provider and discussions with a qualified Pilates instructor. The goal is to map out a clear picture of what your body can handle, pinpoint areas that need special attention, and identify any health conditions that could affect your practice. For instance, knowing that you have reduced bone density could lead your instructor to modify specific exercises to prevent undue strain on your bones.

Customization and Adaptation

Once your physical landscape is understood, the next step is customizing your Pilates regimen. Here, the magic of Pilates truly shines – its inherent flexibility allows for endless adaptations. For seniors dealing with arthritis, for example, exercises can be adjusted to minimize joint stress while still strengthening the muscles around the joints. Similarly, those with osteoporosis might focus on routines that improve balance and coordination, reducing the risk of falls while avoiding high-impact moves that could jeopardize bone health.

- **Arthritis:** The focus shifts to increasing joint mobility and reducing stiffness for tender and inflamed joints. Movements are modified to be gentler, often incorporating props like soft balls or foam rollers to achieve a full range of motion without pain.

•**Osteoporosis:** With the risk of fractures a concern, Pilates for osteoporosis prioritizes exercises that foster balance and build bone density. Weight-bearing exercises performed with care can stimulate bone strengthening, all while ensuring safety is paramount.

•**Back Pain:** Chronic back pain, a common ailment among seniors, requires carefully selecting Pilates exercises that strengthen the core - the abdominal and back muscles - to provide better support for the spine. These routines are designed to be therapeutic, offering relief from discomfort while improving posture.

Listening to Your Body

An integral part of practicing Pilates, especially for seniors, is developing an acute awareness of one's body's signals. This awareness is your safeguard against injury and guide to a fulfilling practice. It involves recognizing the difference between the natural effort involved in Pilates and the pain that signals a problem, understanding when to push a little further and when to pull back. This skill, honed over time, ensures that each session contributes positively to your health without harming you.

For instance, feeling a gentle stretch in your muscles during an exercise is normal and indicative of the work your body is doing. However, if that stretch shifts into sharp pain or discomfort, it's a clear signal from your body to stop and reassess. Recognizing and respecting these signals is non-negotiable in maintaining a healthy Pilates practice.

The Role of Professional Guidance

The value of professional guidance in Pilates for seniors cannot be overstated. Working with an instructor who understands Pilates and the nuances of instructing seniors is vital to safe and effective practice. These professionals can provide the necessary adaptations for your exercises, offer real-time feedback on your form and technique, and help you navigate the challenges unique to your body's condition.

A qualified instructor brings knowledge about Pilates and its interaction with aging bodies. They can foresee potential problems and preemptively adjust your routine, ensuring each movement serves your body's best interests. Moreover, they can act as motivators, helping you set realistic goals and celebrating with you as you achieve them, big or small.

For seniors venturing into Pilates, this professional guidance is more than just a luxury; it's a critical component of the practice. It ensures that Pilates remains a source of strength and vitality, tailored precisely to meet your body's needs and to support your health and well-being as you age.

Navigating the journey of Pilates as a senior is an exercise in balance itself – balancing the eagerness to improve physical fitness with the wisdom to recognize and adapt to your body's limits. Through individual assessments, tailored exercises, attentive body listening, and the support of experienced instructors, Pilates can be a safe, enjoyable, and profoundly beneficial part of aging. It's an invitation to seniors to explore their physical capabilities, to challenge themselves within safe boundaries, and to discover the joy of movement in a way that respects and celebrates their bodies' journey through life.

1.7 THE BENEFITS OF PILATES ON MENTAL HEALTH FOR SENIORS

Maintaining mental health becomes as crucial as physical health in the golden years. Pilates, often praised for its physical benefits, also profoundly impacts mental well-being, offering seniors a holistic approach to health.

Enhancing Emotional Well-being

Pilates has a unique way of nurturing the mind. The practice, with its rhythmic movements and focused breathing, acts as a form of meditation, allowing for a break from the hustle of daily life and the stress it brings. This mindfulness aspect helps lower cortisol levels, the body's primary stress hormone, promoting a state of calmness and relaxation. For many seniors, this reduction in stress and anxiety can be transformative. It offers a respite, a moment of tranquility in their day that can improve overall mood and emotional resilience. The controlled movements and breathing techniques taught in Pilates encourage a state of mental clarity and calm, reducing feelings of anxiety and fostering a sense of peace.

Moreover, mastering new movements and progressing in strength and flexibility contribute to a sense of accomplishment. This, in turn, boosts self-esteem and fosters a positive mood, counteracting feelings of sadness or depression that sometimes accompany aging.

Improving Sleep Quality

The link between Pilates and better sleep is undeniable. The physical exertion involved in Pilates, even though low impact, tires the body well, preparing it for rest. The emphasis on breath control and mindfulness also plays a significant role. It helps quiet the mind, making it easier to fall asleep and stay asleep throughout the night. Improved sleep has a ripple effect on health, enhancing immune function, reducing the risk of chronic diseases, and promoting recovery. Pilates can be a natural remedy for seniors who often struggle with sleep issues, improving the quality of their rest and, by extension, their overall vitality and energy levels.

Social Engagement and Community

Participating in group Pilates classes offer more than just physical benefits; it fosters a sense of community and belonging. For seniors, this social aspect is invaluable. It provides an opportunity to connect with others, share experiences, and enjoy camaraderie. These connections can significantly combat feelings of isolation or loneliness, which are common in later life. The supportive environment of a Pilates class encourages mutual encouragement and the sharing of laughter and joy, contributing to a more prosperous, more fulfilling social life.

The structure of group classes also adds a consistent social event to look forward to each week, providing a routine that can be comforting and stabilizing. This regular social interaction can form solid friendships, enrich seniors' social networks and contribute to their emotional well-being.

Cultivating a Positive Self-image

Pilates aids seniors in developing a more positive self-image. As physical strength and flexibility improve, so does the perception of one's body. This newfound appreciation for what their body can achieve fosters a positive body image and boosts confidence. For many seniors, seeing progress in their Pilates practice, such as reaching a bit further or holding a pose a bit longer, translates into more incredible pride and satisfaction with their bodies.

Moreover, the focus on posture and alignment in Pilates enhances physical appearance. It contributes to a sense of grace and poise. This can change how seniors view themselves and others, leading to a more positive self-image and increased self-esteem. The empowerment from gaining physical strength and flexibility, combined with the mental clarity and calmness fostered by Pilates, contributes to a more holistic sense of self-worth and body positivity.

The benefits of Pilates on mental health for seniors are clear. Through enhancing emotional well-being, improving sleep quality, fostering social engagement, and cultivating a positive self-image, Pilates offers a comprehensive approach to health that addresses seniors' unique challenges. This holistic impact of Pilates goes beyond physical fitness, touching every aspect of life and contributing to a happier, more balanced state of mind.

1.8 SAFETY FIRST: PREVENTING INJURY WITH PROPER TECHNIQUE

Practicing Pilates, particularly for seniors, demands an unwavering commitment to safety to maximize benefits while minimizing the risk of injury. The foundation of this safe practice lies in the proper technique. Precision in movement, one of the core principles of Pilates, isn't just about effectiveness; it's fundamentally about safety. Correct posture and alignment ensure that stress is distributed evenly across the body, preventing undue strain on any part.

For seniors, the stakes are even higher due to the natural vulnerabilities that come with aging, such as reduced bone density and joint flexibility. Therefore, learning the correct way to perform Pilates exercises becomes beneficial and crucial. It begins with mastering the basics, such as engaging the core, aligning the spine, and breathing during exercises. These fundamentals form a protective barrier against common mistakes that could lead to injuries like muscle strains or joint stress.

Proper technique extends beyond the execution of movements to include the setup for each exercise. For instance, it is essential to ensure that the mat or equipment is positioned correctly and that any props used suit the exercise. Though seemingly minor, these preparatory steps play a significant role in creating a safe exercise environment.

Adapting Exercises for Safety

Adapting Pilates exercises for safety is particularly important for seniors with pre-existing health issues or mobility limitations. The versatility of Pilates allows for such adaptations without diminishing the workout's effectiveness. Here are some specific adaptations that can enhance safety:

- **Modifying Positions:** For those with balance issues, exercises can be modified from a standing to a seated or lying position to reduce the risk of falls.
- **Using Props:** Props like chairs for balance, cushions for support, and resistance bands for gentle strengthening can make exercises safer and more accessible.
- **Reducing Range of Motion:** Limiting the range of motion in specific exercises can help avoid overextension and protect vulnerable joints.

These adaptations ensure seniors can participate in Pilates safely, regardless of physical limitations. The key is to tailor the exercises to individual capabilities, ensuring that each movement is performed within a safe range that does not exacerbate existing conditions.

Role of Instructors in Ensuring Safety

Instructors' role in ensuring seniors' safety during Pilates cannot be overstated. A qualified instructor with experience in teaching seniors is invaluable. They possess the knowledge to modify exercises, the insight to identify potential risks, and the skill to tailor sessions to the unique needs of each participant.

Instructors are instrumental in teaching the proper technique, providing immediate feedback on the correct form, and preventing the development of unsafe habits. They can recognize when an exercise is too challenging or potentially harmful and can offer alternatives that maintain the integrity of the workout while ensuring the participant's safety.

Furthermore, instructors can be an educational resource, sharing knowledge about the body's mechanics and how to listen to and interpret its signals. This education empowers seniors to practice Pilates with an awareness that safeguards against injury.

Pre-Exercise Health Screening

Before starting a Pilates regimen, a comprehensive health screening is crucial for identifying potential risks and ensuring that exercises are performed safely. This screening should include an assessment of physical health, including any pre-existing conditions, medications that might affect physical activity, and any limitations or concerns that need to be considered.

A thorough health screening provides valuable information that can be used to adapt Pilates exercises for safety. It highlights areas of concern, such as weakened bones or vulnerable joints, that require special attention during workouts. This proactive approach allows for a customized Pilates experience that maximizes benefits while minimizing risks.

The health screening should be a collaborative process involving the senior, their healthcare provider, and their Pilates instructor. This team approach ensures that all aspects of the senior's health are considered in creating their Pilates regimen, providing a solid foundation for a safe and effective practice.

In Pilates, as in life, safety precedes everything else. For seniors, this means taking the necessary steps to ensure that their Pilates practice is beneficial and safe. From mastering the proper technique and adapting exercises for individual needs to the crucial roles of instructors and pre-exercise health screenings, safety is woven into every aspect of Pilates for seniors. This comprehensive approach to safety supports seniors in their pursuit of fitness, empowering them to enjoy the myriad benefits of Pilates without the shadow of injury. By prioritizing safety, seniors can confidently engage in Pilates, knowing that their well-being is safeguarded, allowing them to focus on the joys and benefits of their practice.

1.9 ADAPTING PILATES FOR VARIOUS SENIOR FITNESS LEVELS

With its inherent flexibility and adaptability, Pilates caters to a wide range of fitness levels, from those taking their first steps into a more active lifestyle to seasoned practitioners looking to deepen their practice. Tailoring Pilates to meet individual needs ensures that everyone can enjoy and benefit from this exercise regardless of their fitness background.

Assessing Fitness Levels

The first step in personalizing a Pilates program involves carefully assessing one's fitness level. This assessment can be conducted by a certified Pilates instructor or a physiotherapist and typically looks at several key areas: flexibility, core strength, balance, and overall mobility. It might also take into account any specific health concerns or physical limitations. This evaluation forms the basis for a tailored Pilates regimen that aligns with individual capabilities and goals, ensuring exercises are both safe and challenging.

Modifications for Beginners

For seniors new to Pilates, modifications to standard exercises help make the practice accessible and enjoyable, laying a solid foundation for their Pilates journey. Here are a few examples of how typical Pilates exercises can be adapted for beginners:

•**Chair-Assisted Squats:** Instead of performing traditional squats that can be challenging for those with knee issues or poor balance, chair-assisted squats offer a supportive way to build leg strength. Standing in front of a chair and slowly lowering the body until it's just above the seat before standing up again provides a safe way to engage the leg muscles without strain.

•**Modified Plank:** For those not ready to perform a full plank, a modified version on the forearms can be done either on the knees or standing and leaning against a wall. This variation still engages the core muscles effectively but with less pressure on the arms and shoulders.

•**Seated Leg Lifts:** Sitting leg lifts can be performed on a chair to build core strength without needing floor exercises. Sitting upright with feet flat on the floor, one leg at a time is lifted and held for a few seconds, engaging the abdominal muscles.

These modifications ensure beginners can gradually build their strength and flexibility, reducing the risk of injury and promoting a positive Pilates experience.

Challenges for Advanced Practitioners

For seniors who have been practicing Pilates for some time and seek to deepen their practice, introducing new challenges keeps the workouts engaging and ensures continued progress. Here are ways to increase the intensity and complexity of Pilates exercises for more advanced practitioners:

- **Incorporate Props:** Adding resistance bands, Pilates rings, or weighted balls can intensify many standard Pilates exercises. For example, holding a Pilates ring between the hands during arm exercises adds an extra layer of resistance, strengthening the upper body more effectively.
- **Increase Repetitions or Hold Times:** Simply increasing the number of repetitions or the length of time each pose is held can significantly enhance the challenge of an exercise. This method requires no additional equipment but effectively builds strength and endurance.
- **Try Advanced Poses:** For those who are ready, advanced Pilates poses like the Teaser or the Jackknife offer a higher difficulty level, engaging the core muscles intensely and improving balance and coordination.

Introducing these challenges maintains an interest in the practice. It ensures that Pilates' benefits continue accumulating, contributing to greater strength, flexibility, and well-being.

Balancing Flexibility, Strength, and Endurance

Creating a balanced Pilates workout involves incorporating exercises that improve flexibility, build strength, and enhance endurance. This holistic approach ensures a well-rounded fitness regimen that addresses all aspects of physical health. Here are strategies for achieving this balance:

- **Combine Dynamic and Static Exercises:** Dynamic exercises like Pilates roll-ups or leg circles improve flexibility and range of motion, while static poses that require holding a position, such as a plank, build strength and endurance.

•**Focus on the Core:** Core-strengthening exercises are central to Pilates and are the foundation for improving strength and flexibility. Exercises like the Hundred or the Double Leg Stretch engage the core muscles and enhance stamina.

•**Incorporate Flowing Sequences:** Flowing sequences that transition smoothly from one pose to another challenge the cardiovascular system, building endurance. These sequences also promote flexibility as the body moves through a full range of motion.

A well-structured Pilates session that includes a mix of these elements ensures that seniors enjoy a varied and engaging workout and reap the full spectrum of benefits Pilates has to offer. By adapting exercises to individual fitness levels and focusing on building flexibility, strength, and endurance, seniors can enhance their physical health and enjoy greater mobility and vitality in their later years.

1.10 PILATES AND CHRONIC CONDITIONS: A GENTLE APPROACH

With its gentle yet effective exercises, Pilates offers hope for seniors navigating the choppy waters of chronic conditions. It stands out for its physical benefits and capacity to alleviate discomfort associated with various chronic ailments, offering a more comfortable and active lifestyle.

Pilates for Arthritis Management

Arthritis, characterized by joint pain and stiffness, significantly impacts the quality of life for many seniors. Pilates, focusing on smooth and controlled movements, emerges as an ideal exercise regimen for managing these symptoms. The gentle stretching and strengthening exercises inherent in Pilates can enhance joint mobility and alleviate pain. For instance, emphasizing low-impact movements helps maintain joint health without the strain that other high-impact activities might impose. Moreover, Pilates strengthens the muscles surrounding the joints, providing them with better support and reducing their burden, which can decrease arthritis-related discomfort.

Supported by Research

The effectiveness of Pilates in managing chronic conditions is more than merely anecdotal. Still, it is supported by a growing body of research. Studies have demonstrated significant benefits of Pilates for individuals suffering from osteoporosis and chronic back pain. One study pointed out that participants engaging in regular Pilates exercises experienced increased bone density, an essential factor in combating osteoporosis. Another research found that individuals with chronic lower back pain who participated in Pilates sessions reported decreased pain levels and an improved range of motion. These findings underscore the potential of Pilates to act as a therapeutic tool in managing and mitigating the impact of chronic conditions on seniors' lives.

Pilates for Cardiovascular Health

Heart disease remains a leading cause of morbidity among seniors, making cardiovascular health a priority. Pilates contributes positively to heart health by promoting physical activity in a manner that is both accessible and sustainable for seniors. Controlled breathing, which is a staple of Pilates, plays a crucial role in this regard. It encourages better oxygenation of the blood and improves circulation, both vital components of cardiovascular health. Moreover, the stress-reducing effects of Pilates can lower blood pressure, a significant risk factor for heart disease. By integrating Pilates into their weekly routines, seniors can take a proactive step towards maintaining a healthy heart and preventing the onset of heart disease.

Guidance for Practicing with Chronic Conditions

For seniors with chronic conditions eager to explore the benefits of Pilates, proceeding with caution and mindfulness is key. Here are some practical tips for safely incorporating Pilates into their routine:

- **Consult with Healthcare Providers:** Before starting Pilates or any new exercise regimen, seniors should consult their healthcare providers. This step is crucial for ensuring Pilates is safe for their specific health conditions.
- **Work with Qualified Instructors:** Finding an instructor who is experienced in working with seniors and knowledgeable about modifications for various chronic conditions can make all the difference.

These professionals can tailor exercises to meet individual needs, ensuring safety and maximizing benefits.

• **Start Slow:** Gradually easing into Pilates allows the body to adjust to new movements and challenges without overwhelming it. Beginning with basic exercises and slowly progressing ensures a safe and enjoyable experience.

• **Monitor Your Body's Response:** Paying close attention to how the body responds during and after Pilates sessions is vital. Any sign of discomfort or pain should be taken seriously, and exercises should be adjusted accordingly.

• **Stay Consistent:** Regularity is key in Pilates, especially for managing chronic conditions. Consistent practice amplifies the benefits, helping seniors see gradual improvements in their condition and overall well-being.

• **Embrace Modifications:** There's no one-size-fits-all in Pilates, especially for those with chronic conditions. Embracing modifications and using props when necessary can help personalize the practice to one's abilities and limitations, making it more effective and enjoyable.

Following these guidelines can help seniors with chronic conditions safely enjoy the benefits of Pilates, turning it into a supportive pillar in their quest for a healthier, more active life. Pilates offers a path that balances physical activity with inner calm, promoting well-being in a holistic, accessible, and sustainable manner.

2

GENTLE WALL PILATES FOR SENIORS: BUILDING STRENGTH AND STABILITY

Imagine a tool so versatile and supportive that it's almost as if you had a personal Pilates instructor at home with you. Look around; it might be leaning against your living room or bedroom wall. We're talking about that unassuming, solid surface you've walked by countless times. The wall, an ever-present feature in our homes, is about to become your steadfast ally in practicing Pilates. With it, you'll discover new ways to enhance strength, balance, and flexibility, catering specifically to your needs as a senior.

Wall Pilates strips away the intimidation factor of traditional Pilates mat exercises, making the practice approachable for everyone. It's about using what's already there in your home to support your fitness journey. This section dives into how the wall can be your partner in building a stronger, more balanced you.

Leveraging the Wall for Support

The beauty of using the wall for Pilates exercises lies in its stability. Here's why that's important:

• **Prevents Falls:** For seniors, maintaining balance during exercise is crucial. The wall acts as a sturdy prop, minimizing the risk of falls during routines.

- **Increases Confidence:** Knowing you have support allows you to attempt exercises that might otherwise seem daunting, gradually building your confidence in your physical abilities.
- **Enhances Focus:** With the wall as your support, you can concentrate better on mastering the form and breathing techniques essential to Pilates rather than worrying about maintaining balance.

2.1 BASIC WALL EXERCISES

- **Wall Rolls:** Stand with your back against the wall, feet hip-width apart. Slowly roll down, vertebra by vertebra, keeping your lower back in contact with the wall. Roll down as far as comfortable, then slowly roll back up. This exercise warms up your spine and engages your core.

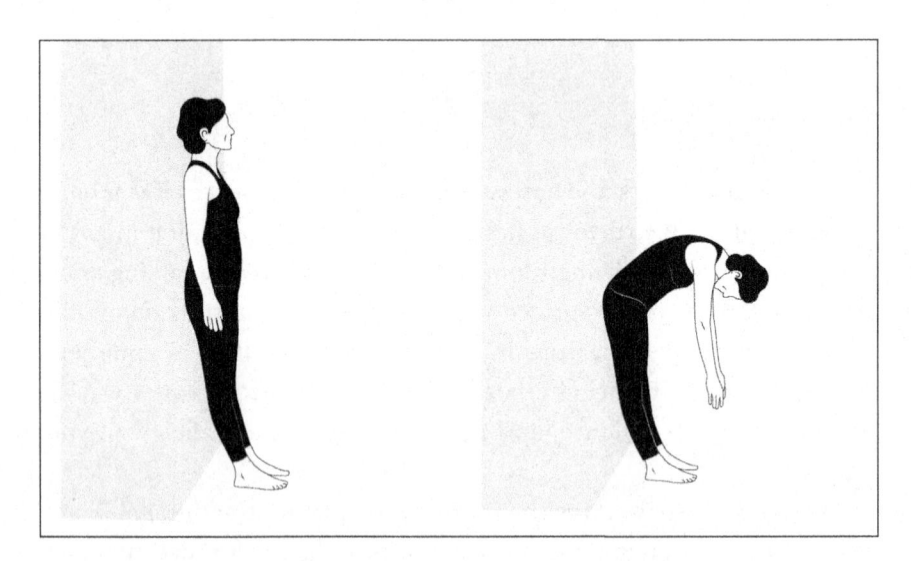

- **Alternate Leg Slides:** Lean against the wall with your arms by your sides. Keep one leg grounded for support and slide the other leg up and down the wall in a controlled manner. The slow and deliberate movement focuses on maintaining continuous contact between the leg and the wall, which helps stabilize the body and engage the core and leg muscles effectively. This exercise emphasizes precision and balance, which are core to Pilates practice, ensuring that the practitioner maintains proper alignment and engagement throughout the movement.

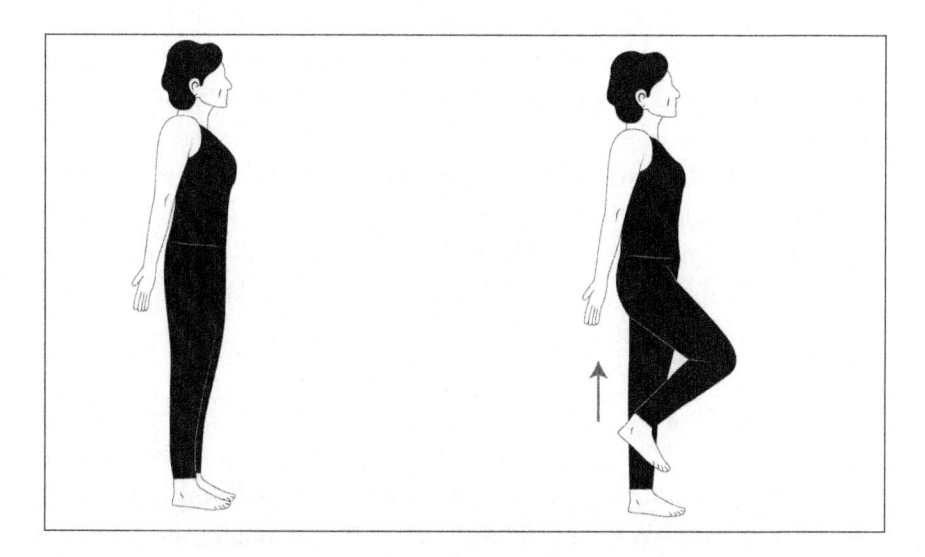

These exercises are just the starting point. They focus on engaging your core and improving balance without putting undue stress on your body.

Progressions and Modifications

As you become more comfortable and your strength increases, consider ways to add variety and challenge to your wall Pilates exercises:

• **Increase Range of Motion:** Gradually increase how far you slide your leg or how low you roll down the wall. Always listen to your body, ensuring you're challenging but not straining yourself.

• **Add Resistance:** Introduce light resistance bands to exercises like leg slides for an added strength component.

• **Incorporate Balance Challenges:** As your confidence grows, lift one foot off the ground slightly during wall rolls to further challenge your balance.

For those with specific health conditions, modifications ensure exercises remain safe and effective:

• **For Arthritis:** Keep movements smooth and range limited to avoid joint stress. Use cushioning like a soft mat against the wall for comfort.

• **For Osteoporosis:** Avoid twisting motions and focus on stability and gentle stretches.

Integrating Wall Exercises into Daily Routines

Making wall Pilates a part of your daily life doesn't require carving out large chunks of time. Here's how to seamlessly include these exercises:

• **Morning Routine:** Start your day with a few wall rolls to wake up your spine and get the blood flowing.

• **Break Time:** Incorporate leg slides during TV commercials or while waiting for the kettle to boil. It's a quick way to keep moving and break up periods of sitting.

• **Evening Wind Down:** Before bed, use the wall for gentle stretches, which will help relax your muscles and mind for a good night's sleep.

The wall in your home is more than just structural; it's a tool waiting to be used in your Pilates practice. By leveraging this support, starting with basic exercises and gradually introducing progressions and modifications, you'll build strength, balance, and flexibility safely and effectively. Wall Pilates offers a bridge between the desire to stay active and the challenges that sometimes accompany traditional exercise methods for seniors. It proves that with some creativity, the resources we need to maintain our health and well-being are often right in front of us—or, in this case, right behind us.

2.2 BUILDING CORE STRENGTH WITHOUT THE FLOOR: WALL-BASED EXERCISES

The core of our body, much like the foundation of a house, holds everything together, ensuring stability, strength, and balance. For seniors, maintaining and enhancing core strength is not just beneficial—it's crucial for everyday activities. Yet, the thought of engaging in traditional floor exercises to strengthen the core may seem daunting or even unattainable for some. Enter wall-based Pilates exercises: a game-changer for those who find getting down to or up from the floor challenging. This section unfolds the myriad benefits of wall-supported core strengthening, introduces specific exercises tailored for seniors, and shares safety precautions to ensure a rewarding practice.

Advantages of Wall-Based Core Work

The wall provides an unparalleled support system for performing

Pilates exercises, especially for core strengthening. Here's why it's particularly advantageous:

- **Accessibility:** The wall makes core strengthening exercises more accessible, eliminating the need to lie on the floor. This is especially helpful for those with mobility issues or discomfort when bending.
- **Stability and Safety:** Using the wall for support enhances exercise stability, reducing the risk of falls and injuries. This added safety layer encourages seniors to engage their core muscles more confidently.
- **Focused Engagement:** The resistance provided by the wall allows for a more focused engagement of the core muscles. When pushing against a stable surface, you can isolate and activate the core more effectively.

Key Wall-Based Core Exercises

- **Standing Planks:** Stand an arm's length away from the wall, facing it. Place your palms and forearms on the wall at shoulder height. Step back until your body forms a straight line from head to heels, leaning into the wall. Engage your core and hold this position, breathing deeply. This exercise helps maintain core engagement while offering a supportive, adaptable alternative to the traditional floor plank.

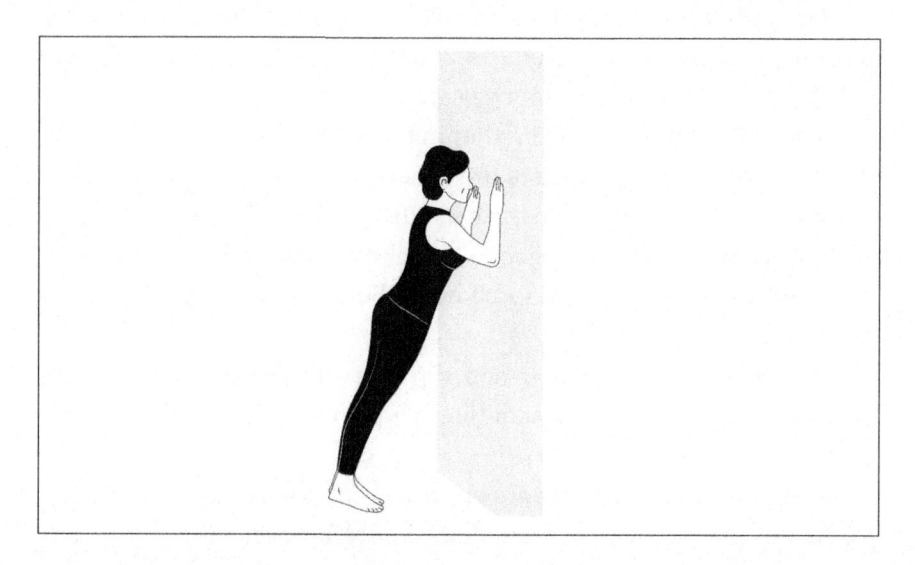

- **Wall Push-ups:** Face the wall, placing your hands on it slightly wider than shoulder-width apart. Step your feet back so your body is at a slight angle. Bend your elbows to lower your chest towards the wall, engaging your core to keep your body straight. Push back to the starting position. The focus is on building upper body strength through this accessible and effective exercise.

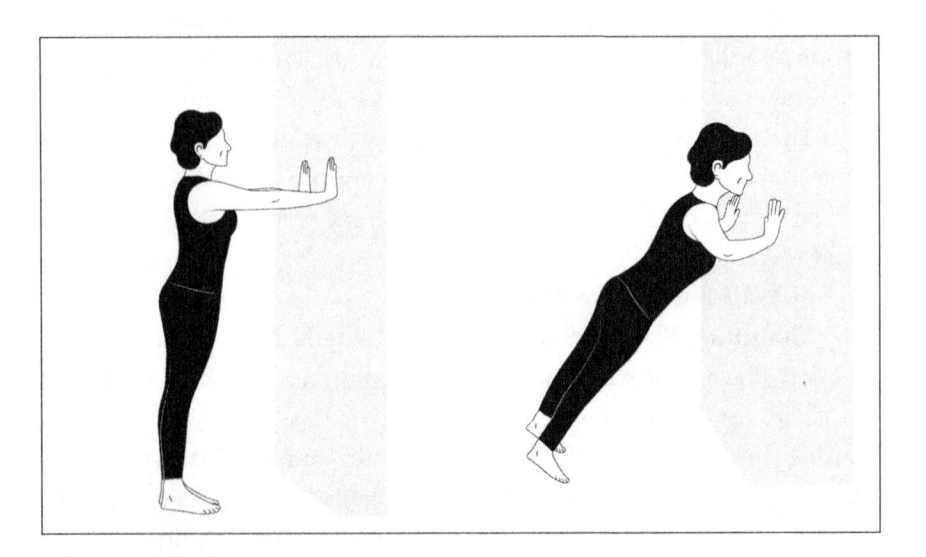

These exercises are pillars for building core strength, enhancing posture, and improving overall stability—critical components for a healthy, active lifestyle in senior years.

Safety Tips for Core Strengthening

While wall-based exercises are inherently safer, observing certain precautions ensures you reap the benefits without risking overexertion:

• **Warm-up:** Begin with gentle stretches or a short walk to prepare your body. This increases blood flow to the muscles, reducing the risk of strains.

• **Proper Footwear:** Wear non-slip shoes to prevent sliding, especially during exercises like standing planks where your feet are your anchor.

• **Alignment Check:** Always ensure your body is correctly aligned. With wall push-ups, your shoulders should be over your wrists, and your body should form a straight line in standing planks. Incorrect alignment can lead to unnecessary strain.

- **Listen to Your Body:** The golden rule of any exercise is to listen to your body. If you experience discomfort or pain, stop and adjust. Your body's signals are paramount in guiding a safe practice.

Customizing Core Workouts

Tailoring your core-strengthening routine is critical to a successful practice, ensuring exercises are challenging yet within your capability:

- **Adjust Distance from the Wall:** Modifying how far you stand from the wall can increase or decrease the difficulty of exercises. Standing closer makes exercises like wall push-ups less challenging and suitable for beginners.
- **Incorporate Variations:** Once you're comfortable, introduce variations. For example, alternate lifting one leg at a time in standing planks to further engage the core.
- **Frequency and Duration:** Start with shorter sessions, gradually increasing as your strength builds. Consistency is more beneficial than intensity in the initial stages.

By integrating these wall-based exercises into your routine, you're working towards a stronger core and investing in your independence, mobility, and quality of life. The wall, an omnipresent feature in our homes, transforms into a tool for empowerment, enabling seniors to engage in Pilates confidently, safely, and effectively. Through these tailored exercises, the journey towards enhanced core strength and stability is not only accessible but also enjoyable, marking a significant step in embracing a holistic approach to health and wellness in the senior years.

2.3 ENHANCING FLEXIBILITY AND RANGE OF MOTION GENTLY

Flexibility is pivotal in our overall health, particularly as we navigate the later years of life. It's not just about being able to touch your toes or reach high shelves; it's about maintaining the range of motion necessary for daily activities and preventing injuries. For seniors, incorporating gentle stretching into their fitness regimen is key to preserving and improving flexibility.

Pilates offers various stretching techniques specifically designed to increase flexibility and range of motion safely. Unlike some forms of exercise that push the body to its limits, Pilates emphasizes gentle, controlled movements that can significantly enhance flexibility without the risk of injury. This approach ensures that stretching becomes a regular part of your routine and a much-anticipated one, thanks to its gentle nature.

Creating a daily routine of Pilates stretches can be a game-changer for seniors looking to maintain or enhance their flexibility. Here's how to build one:

• **Morning Stretch:** Start your day with standing wall slides to wake your muscles gently. This involves standing with your back against the wall and slowly sliding your arms up overhead, keeping contact with the wall. This exercise emphasizes controlled arm motion, enhancing shoulder mobility and stability while engaging the upper back and arm muscles.

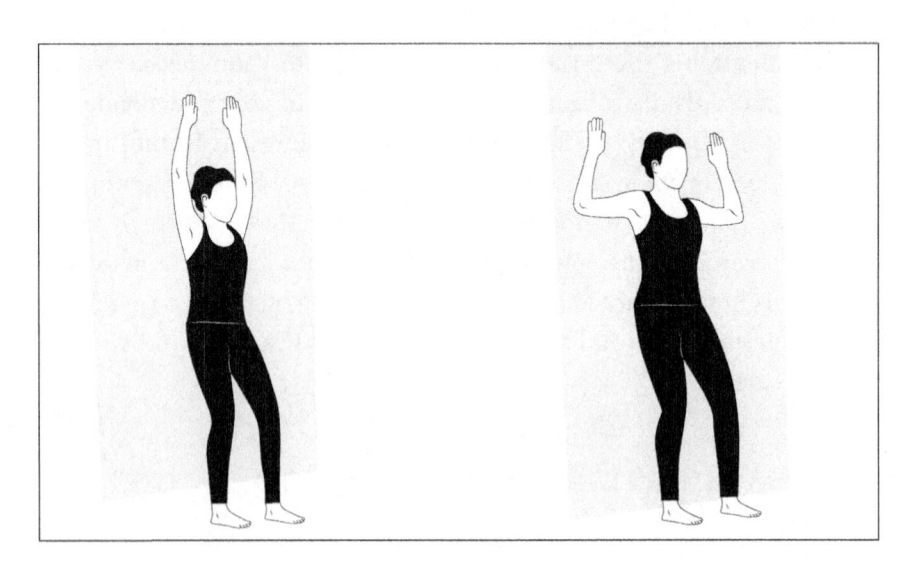

• **Midday Movement:** Incorporate seated leg extensions into your afternoon routine. While sitting in a chair, extend one leg at a time, reaching forward from your hips to feel a stretch along the back of your leg. This is particularly beneficial for loosening tight hamstrings and improving lower back flexibility.

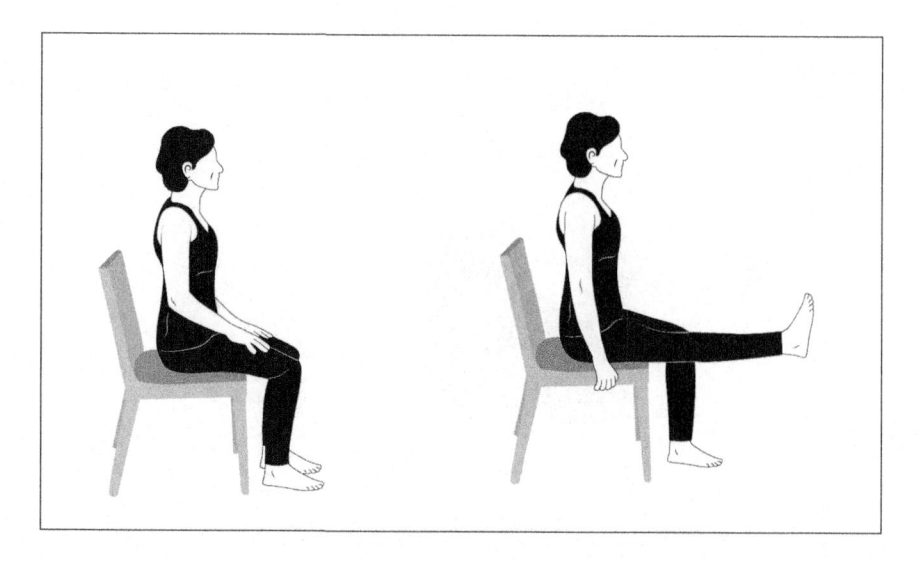

- **Evening Wind-down:** Before bedtime, engage in gentle spine twists to relax your body and ease any tension built up during the day. Sitting on a mat with legs crossed or extended, keep your spine straight and engage your core. Extend your arms to the sides at shoulder level, and rotate your torso to one side, leading with the opposite hand towards the leading knee while your other hand reaches back for a gentle twist. Allow your head to look back towards the twist. This exercise emphasizes controlled rotation, targeting the obliques and improving spinal mobility, all while maintaining a grounded and stable seated posture.

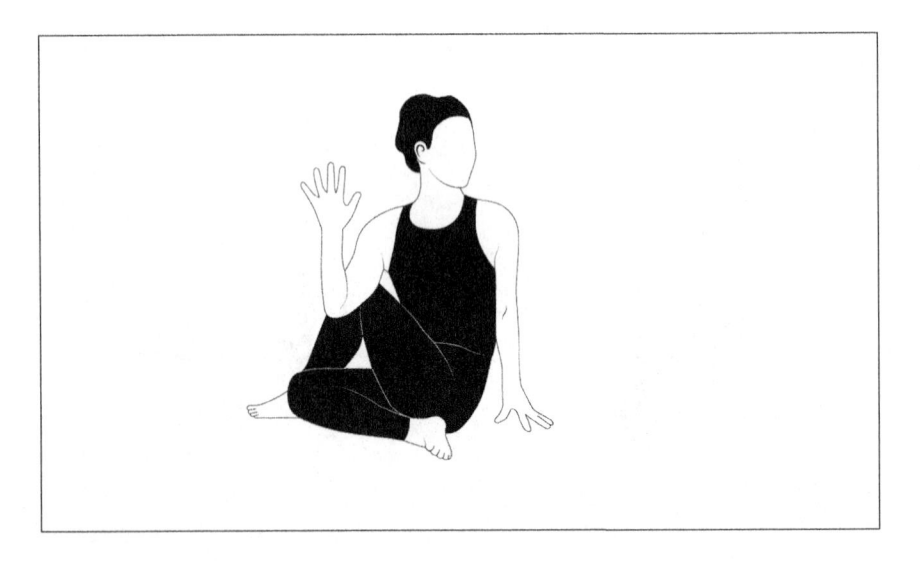

Aim to stretch for at least 10-15 minutes daily for optimal results. The best times to stretch are when your muscles are already warm, such as after a light walk or following your daily activities, to reduce the risk of strains.

Measuring progress in flexibility involves patience and consistency. Unlike strength training, where improvements can be more rapidly observed, increases in flexibility may take longer to manifest. Here's how seniors can track their progress:

• **Keep a Stretching Journal:** Note the stretches you perform each day and any increases in the range of motion you observe. For example, if reaching toward your toes becomes easier over time, record these milestones.

• **Use Visual Aids:** Taking periodic photos or videos of yourself performing stretches can provide visual evidence of your progress. Compare these over time to see how your range of motion has improved.

• **Listen to Your Body:** Paying attention to how you feel can also be a measure of progress. You may notice less stiffness in the mornings or find it easier to perform daily tasks. These qualitative improvements are just as significant as the quantitative ones.

Incorporating gentle Pilates stretching techniques into a daily routine offers seniors a safe and effective way to enhance their flexibility and range of motion. By doing so, they can enjoy a greater degree of independence in their daily activities and significantly reduce their risk of falls and injuries. With patience and consistency, measurable progress will follow, contributing to a higher quality of life and well-being.

2.4 BALANCE AND STABILITY THROUGH WALL PILATES

Navigating daily life safely as we age requires balance and stability, qualities that might wane without mindful attention and care. A decline in these crucial physical attributes can lead to a higher risk of falls and injuries, concerns that are especially pertinent for seniors. Pilates, particularly when practiced with the support of a wall, offers an accessible route to bolstering these essential skills, enhancing one's ability to move through life confidently and safely.

Understanding Balance Challenges

Several factors contribute to challenges with balance and stability in seniors. Diminished muscle strength, vision changes, reduced flexibility, and slower reflexes play a part. Additionally, medications and certain health conditions can impact balance. The good news is that Pilates, with its focus on core strength, flexibility, and mindful movement, can significantly mitigate these issues. By engaging in Pilates exercises that specifically target balance and stability, seniors can improve their proprioception—the body's ability to perceive its position in space—thereby reducing the risk of falls.

Pilates Exercises for Balance

The wall serves as a steadfast partner in several Pilates exercises designed to enhance balance:

- **Single-Leg Stands:** Stand with your side to the wall, lightly touching it with one hand for support. Slowly lift one foot off the ground, maintaining balance on the standing leg. Hold for a few breaths, then switch sides. This exercise hones balance and strengthens the leg muscles.

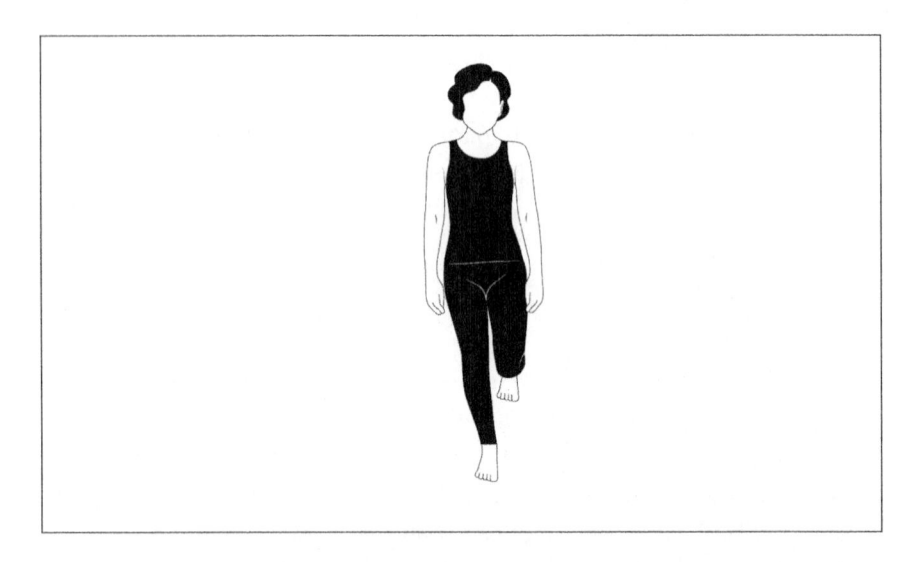

- **Wall Squats:** Face away from the wall, with feet hip-width apart, a step forward. Lean back until your back is flat against the wall. Slide down into a squat position, aiming to get your thighs parallel to the floor, then press back up. This builds lower body strength and stability.

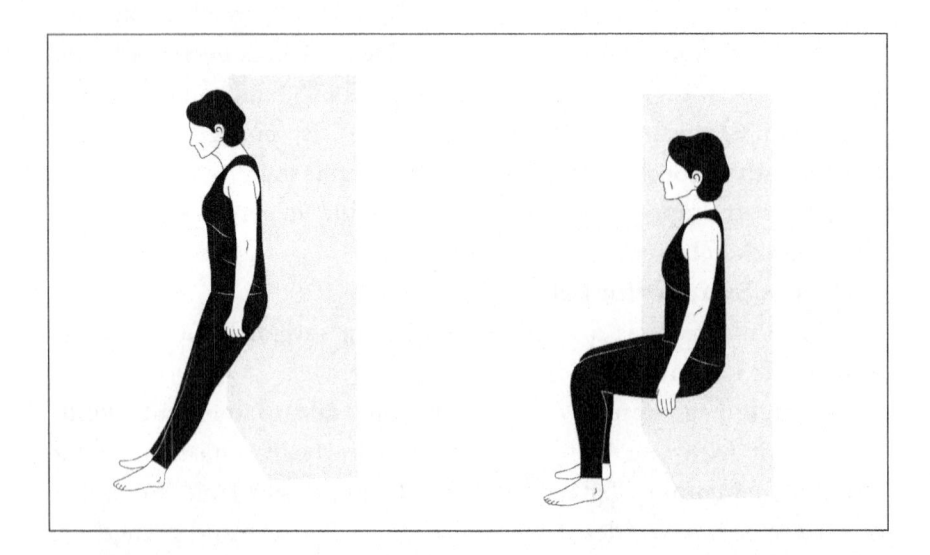

Incorporating these exercises into regular practice targets the muscles essential for balance. It trains the body to maintain stability during various movements, translating to increased safety and confidence in daily activities.

The Role of Core Strength in Stability

At the core (pun intended) of balance and stability lies, well, the core. This muscle group acts as the body's center of gravity, and strengthening it is pivotal for enhancing balance. Wall Pilates exercises, such as the standing plank or wall push-ups, engage and fortify these muscles, providing a solid foundation for stability. A strong core ensures more than good posture; it's instrumental in preventing falls by enabling seniors to recover balance swiftly should they start to trip or stumble.

Creating a Safe Environment

Practicing balance exercises, even with the wall's support, calls for a setup that prioritizes safety:

- **Clear Space**: Ensure the area around your practice space is clutter-free. A clear space minimizes the risk of tripping or bumping into objects if you lose balance momentarily.
- **Appropriate Footwear**: Wear shoes with a good grip to prevent slipping. This is particularly important when practicing standing exercises where a secure footing is essential.
- **Mat Placement**: Positioning a yoga mat or a non-slip mat on the floor where you practice can provide additional safety, offering a soft landing spot for your feet and reducing slip hazards.

By cultivating an environment that encourages safe practice, seniors can confidently engage in their Pilates routine, focusing on improving their balance and stability without the concern of potential accidents.

Seniors can significantly enhance their balance and stability by understanding the nuances of balance challenges, engaging in targeted Pilates exercises, harnessing the power of core strength, and setting up a safe practice environment. This contributes to a reduced risk of falls and empowers seniors to move through their daily lives with greater security and independence. The wall, an ever-present feature in our homes, emerges as a key ally in this pursuit, offering support and resistance that make Pilates an effective tool in the quest for a balanced and stable life.

2.5 BREATHWORK AND PILATES: ENHANCING LUNG CAPACITY AND RELAXATION

Breathing is an automatic process, yet when we bring intentionality to it, especially within the context of Pilates, it becomes transformative. The breath is not just a companion to movement; it's a force that energizes, stabilizes, and revitalizes our body. This holds especially true for seniors, for whom breathwork in Pilates can significantly enhance lung capacity, aid in relaxation, and serve as a vital tool for stress relief.

The Pilates Breathing Technique

The Pilates breathing technique, often called lateral or thoracic breathing, is distinct from the breathing patterns you might encounter in other fitness realms. Rather than inhaling to expand the belly, this method focuses on widening the ribcage sideways without disturbing the engaged core. Here's how it's beneficial:

• **Maximizes Oxygen Intake**: This form of breathing encourages deeper inhalations and more complete exhalations, increasing oxygen intake and enhancing the efficiency of your body's use.

• **Supports Core Stability**: Keeping the abdominals engaged even during breathwork reinforces core stability, which is crucial for balance and posture.

For seniors, mastering this breathing technique can improve respiratory function, which is vital for maintaining active lifestyles and promoting overall health.

Exercises to Improve Lung Capacity

Certain Pilates exercises specifically aim to improve lung capacity by incorporating mindful thoracic breathing. For example:

• **Seated Spine Stretch**: Sit tall with legs extended and arms reaching forward. As you exhale, reach further, curving your spine into a 'C' shape, focusing on expanding the ribcage sideways as you breathe. This stretches the spine and challenges you to maintain deep, controlled breaths.

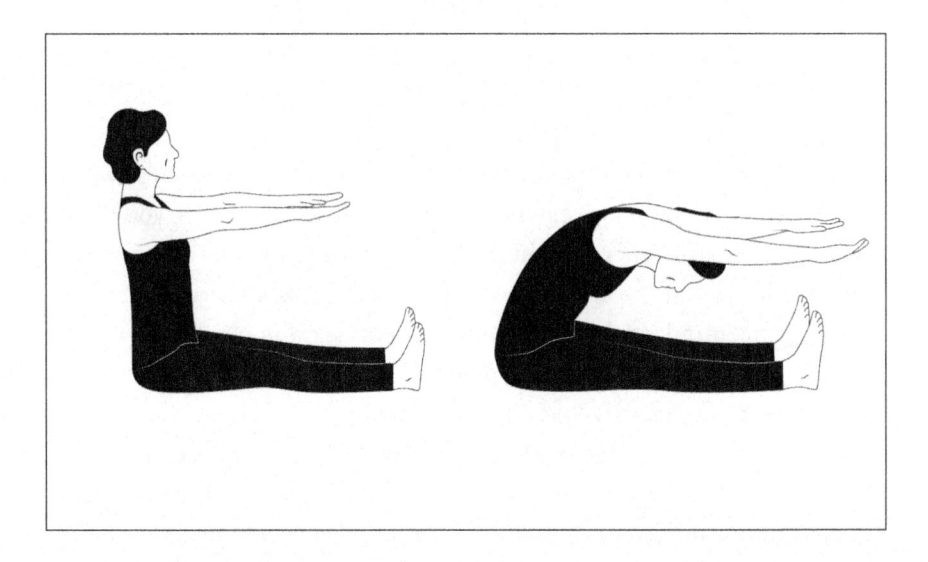

- **The Saw:** Sit with legs wide apart, arms extended out to the sides. Twist your torso to one side, and as you exhale, reach your opposite hand to your foot, looking behind you. This exercise encourages deep breaths while twisting, opening the ribcage, and enhancing lung capacity.

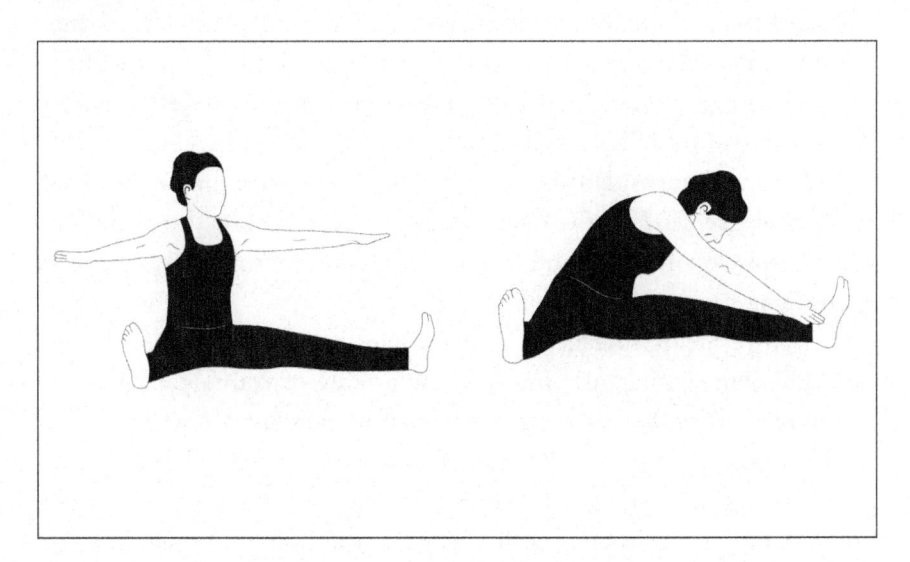

Incorporating these exercises into your routine can progressively enhance your lung function, making activities of daily living easier and more enjoyable.

Breathwork for Stress Relief

The focused breathing involved in Pilates doubles as a powerful tool for stress relief. Concentrating on the breath can shift your body out of the stress-induced 'fight or flight' mode and into a calm state. The rhythmic nature of Pilates breathwork acts like a meditation, clearing the mind and easing tension. For seniors dealing with the stresses of aging, this aspect of Pilates offers a welcome respite, promoting mental clarity and emotional peace.

- **Practice Deep Breathing:** Even outside of your Pilates exercises, take moments to practice deep, thoracic breathing. This can be especially calming during moments of stress, helping to lower heart rate and blood pressure.
- **Visualization:** Combine your breathwork with visualization to deepen its impact. Imagine inhaling peace and calm and exhaling stress and tension. This mental imagery, paired with breathwork, can significantly amplify the stress-relieving benefits.

Incorporating Breathwork into Everyday Life

The beauty of Pilates breathwork is its applicability beyond the mat. Here are practical ways to weave these techniques into your daily life:

- **Morning Ritual:** Start your day with a few minutes of seated thoracic breathing. This sets a calm, centered tone for the day ahead.
- **During Chores:** During daily activities like gardening or cooking, remind yourself to breathe deeply using the lateral breathing method. This keeps you relaxed and keeps your core continuously engaged, reinforcing strength and stability.
- **Before Sleep:** Engage in gentle Pilates breathing exercises before bed. This can significantly improve the quality of your sleep, allowing you to relax more deeply and fall asleep more quickly.

Incorporating Pilates breathwork into your everyday life enhances physical health by improving lung capacity, encouraging relaxation, and serving as a cornerstone for mental well-being. For seniors, this holistic approach to wellness, centered around the power of breath, can mark a significant shift towards a more vibrant, serene, and balanced lifestyle. Through these practices, breathing transforms into an art form that nourishes the body, calms the mind, and enriches the soul, proving that the essence of vitality lies within the breath itself.

2.6 TAILORING PILATES TO ADDRESS LOWER BACK PAIN

Lower back pain is a common ailment troubling many seniors, affecting their daily activities and quality of life. Pilates is a gentle yet effective exercise to manage and alleviate this discomfort. Its systematic approach focuses on strengthening core muscles and improving spinal alignment, which is pivotal in mitigating lower back issues.

Pilates' Approach to Managing Back Pain

Pilates zeroes in on the core, not merely as a way to achieve flat abs but as a method to provide robust support for the entire back. Strengthening these core muscles is a supportive brace for your lower back, easing pressure and pain. Moreover, Pilates emphasizes spinal alignment and controlled, precise movements that enhance posture and flexibility, further relieving back pain. This dual focus on strength and alignment underpins Pilates' effectiveness in addressing lower back pain.

Safe Exercises for Back Pain Relief

Select Pilates exercises are beneficial for strengthening the lower back and alleviating pain. These include:

- **Pelvic Tilts:** Lying on your back with knees bent, gently tilt your pelvis up towards your belly button, pressing your lower back into the floor. This simple movement increases lumbar mobility and strengthens the abdominal muscles that support the lower back.

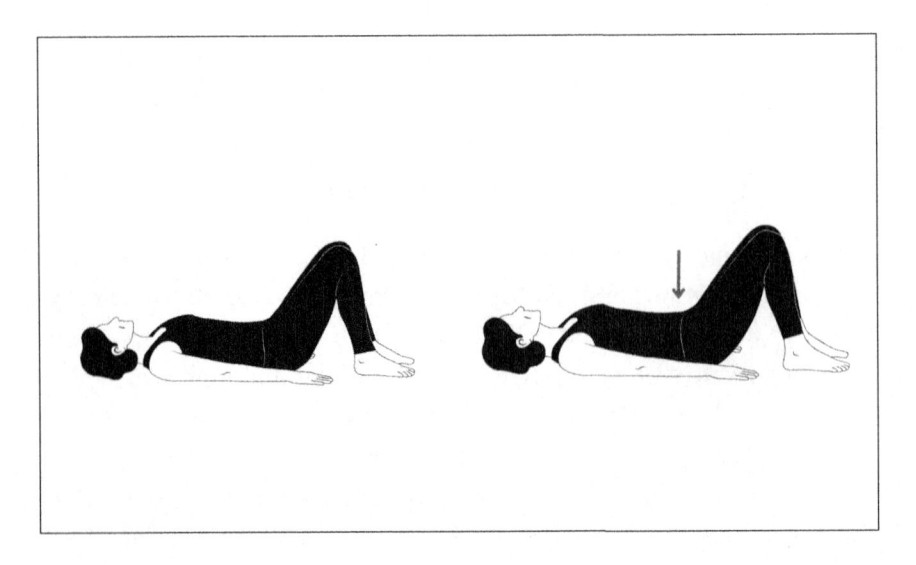

- **Chest Lifts**: From the same starting position, lift your head and chest gently off the floor, keeping your lower back pressed down. This exercise targets the upper abdominal muscles, reducing strain on the lower back.

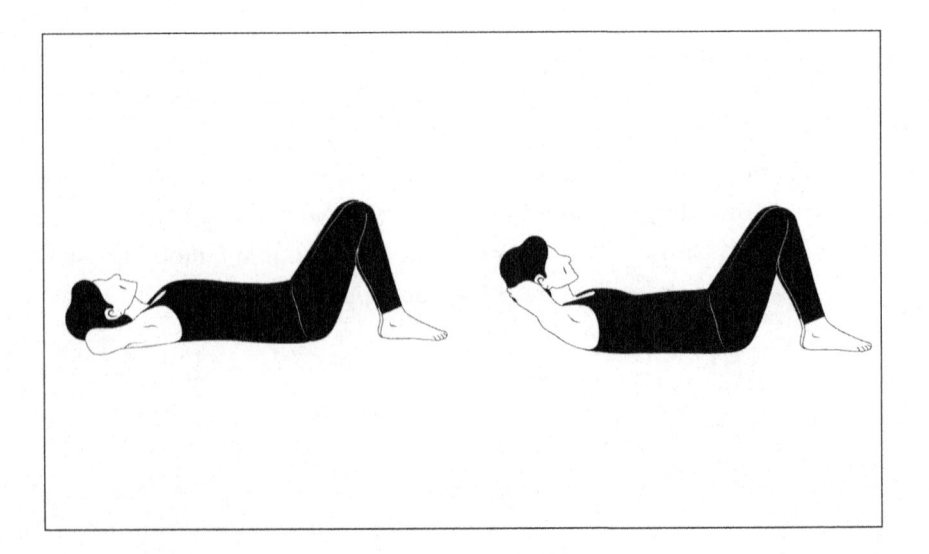

Modifications ensure these exercises remain accessible and beneficial:

- **Use of Props**: Placing a small, folded towel under the lower back during pelvic tilts can provide additional support and comfort.
- **Reduced Range of Motion**: For chest lifts, keeping the range of motion small ensures the focus remains on engaging the core without straining the back.

Avoiding Common Mistakes

Awareness of certain pitfalls is key to practicing Pilates for back pain relief safely:

- **Overarching the Back**: Especially in exercises like the chest lift, there's a tendency to arch the back excessively. Maintaining a neutral spine protects against exacerbating back pain.
- **Straining the Neck**: Lifting the head and shoulders should engage the core, not strain the neck. Keeping the gaze upwards and a slight space under the chin can prevent neck strain.

Consultation with Health Professionals

Before incorporating Pilates into your routine for back pain management, a consultation with healthcare professionals is imperative. This step ensures that Pilates exercises suit your specific condition and that you're aware of any movements to avoid. A healthcare provider can offer insights into the root cause of your back pain, which is critical in tailoring Pilates exercises to your needs. Armed with this information, you can approach Pilates in a way that safeguards against further injury and maximizes each movement's healing and strengthening potential.

Incorporating Pilates into a routine to manage lower back pain offers a path toward relief and a stronger, more resilient back. Pilates can significantly improve the quality of life for seniors dealing with back pain by combining core strengthening, posture enhancement, and flexibility exercises tailored to safety and individual needs. This approach, grounded in understanding and respecting the body's limits and potential, underscores Pilates' role as a powerful tool in maintaining and recovering back health.

2.7 PILATES MOVEMENTS FOR IMPROVING POSTURE IN SENIORS

Good posture is the backbone of not only how we carry ourselves but also how we perform daily activities with ease and efficiency. For seniors, maintaining an upright posture goes beyond aesthetics; it prevents pain, enhances breathing, and improves balance. Pilates, with its core-centered exercises, is pivotal in reinforcing postural alignment. It teaches the body to engage the right muscles for standing tall, effectively distributing weight, and minimizing strain on any single part of the body.

- **Direct Benefits:** Pilates exercises encourage strengthening the core and back muscles, which are essential to good posture. By focusing on these muscle groups, seniors can counteract common postural issues such as rounded shoulders and forward head posture, often exacerbated by lifestyle factors like prolonged sitting.

Posture-Improving Exercises

A few targeted Pilates movements can make significant strides in improving posture. Each exercise focuses on alignment, strength, and flexibility, creating a well-rounded approach to better posture.

- **Chest Expansion:** This exercise requires standing tall, feet hip-width apart, with your back lightly touching the wall. Cross your arms in front of you, then open your arms slowly until your palms touch the wall. Press slightly against the wall, hold for a few seconds, then repeat. The movement encourages shoulder retraction and engagement of the upper back muscles, countering the tendency to slump forward.

GENTLE WALL PILATES FOR SENIORS:

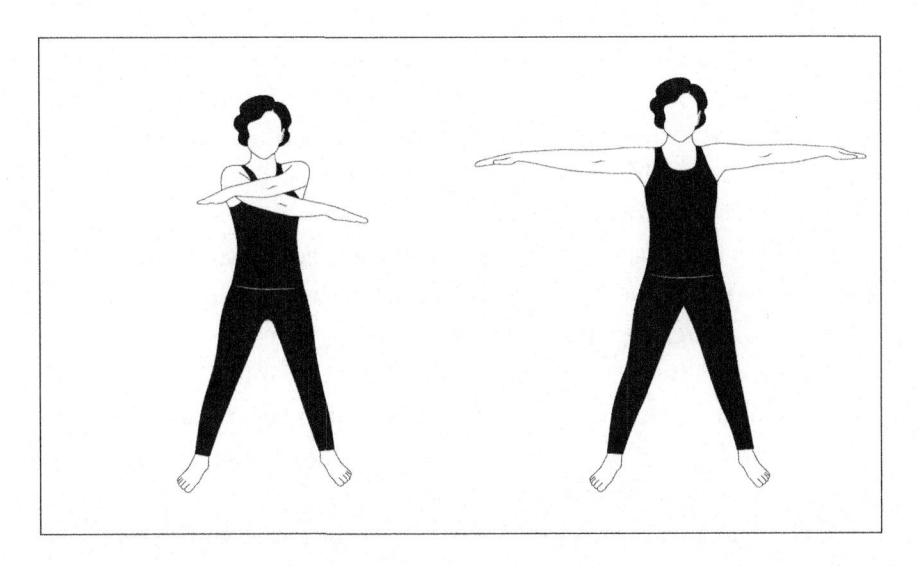

- **Pilates Mermaid:** Sitting on a chair or the floor, place one hand on the seat and reach the other arm up and over your head, creating a side stretch. This movement stretches the side body and helps realign the spine, promoting a straighter posture and enhancing lateral flexibility.

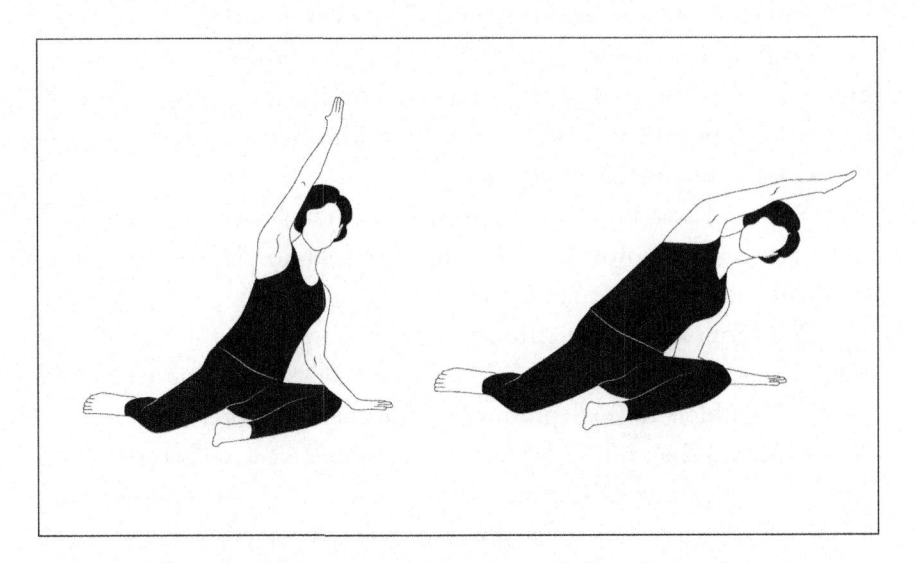

- **Spine Stretch Forward:** Sitting tall on the edge of a chair with legs slightly apart, extend your arms in front of you at shoulder height.

Inhale to prepare, and as you exhale, reach forward, allowing your head to follow the movement of your arms, curving your spine into a gentle 'C' shape. This exercise stretches the spine, encourages flexibility, and engages the abdominal muscles, which support the lower back.

Monitoring Posture Progress

Tracking improvements in posture involves both visual and physical cues. Here are ways seniors can observe advancements in their postural alignment through regular Pilates practice:

- **Mirror Check:** Periodically standing side-on to a full-length mirror to observe posture can reveal gradual changes. Look for a reduction in rounding of the shoulders, a more naturally aligned head position, and a slight curve in the lower back.
- **Physical Markers:** Improvement in posture often translates to less back and neck pain due to better alignment. Increased ease when performing daily activities, from walking to reaching overhead, also indicates progress.
- **Clothing Fit:** Sometimes, how clothes fit can hint at postural changes. Shirts might hang differently, with less pulling across the shoulders, indicating reduced rounding.

Incorporating Posture Awareness in Daily Activities

Bringing the principles of Pilates into everyday life ensures the benefits extend beyond practice sessions. Maintaining posture awareness throughout the day can transform routine activities into opportunities for reinforcing good posture:

- **Sitting:** Use a lumbar support pillow when seated to encourage a slight curve in the lower back. Ensure your feet are flat on the ground and your shoulders are relaxed but not slumped.
- **Walking:** Imagine a string pulling you up from the top of your head as you walk. This visualization helps keep the spine elongated, and the shoulders relaxed, promoting an upright posture.
- **Lifting:** When lifting objects, bend at the knees and keep the back straight, engaging your core muscles. This practice protects your back and reinforces the Pilates principle of core engagement.

Transforming daily habits by integrating posture awareness fundamentally changes how seniors interact with their environment, making every action a conscious step toward improved posture. Pilates offers the tools and techniques to strengthen the body's support system, but applying these principles throughout the day solidifies the posture improvements gained through practice. This holistic approach ensures that the benefits of Pilates extend into every facet of life, allowing seniors to stand taller, move confidently, and live without the limitations imposed by poor posture.

2.8 THE ROLE OF PILATES IN MANAGING ARTHRITIS PAIN

Pilates emerges as a beacon of hope for those grappling with arthritis pain. Its essence lies in gentle, controlled movements that enhance mobility while being kind to the joints. This characteristic makes Pilates a practical, non-pharmacological approach to mitigating the discomfort associated with arthritis.

Arthritis, marked by joint inflammation, leads to pain, stiffness, and decreased range of motion, often hindering daily activities. Pilates, with its core principle of controlled movement, presents a pathway to maintaining and improving joint health and mobility for those suffering from arthritis.

Pilates as a Non-Pharmacological Intervention

Pilates stands out for its adaptability and gentle approach, making it a preferred exercise method for managing arthritis pain. The method's low-impact nature ensures that exercises strengthen without straining, offering relief and enhancing joint mobility. This adaptability allows individuals to maintain an active lifestyle, crucial for effectively managing arthritis symptoms.

Exercises for Joint Health

A selection of Pilates exercises, specifically tailored for individuals with arthritis, focuses on improving joint mobility and reducing stiffness:

- **The Shoulder Bridge:** Lying on your back with knees bent and hip-width apart, place your arms by your side with your palms down. Place one leg straight out, and as you exhale, lift your pelvis and hips until you create a straight line from your knee to your shoulder. Alternate legs. This exercise strengthens the lower back and hips, areas often affected by arthritis, without placing undue stress on the joints.

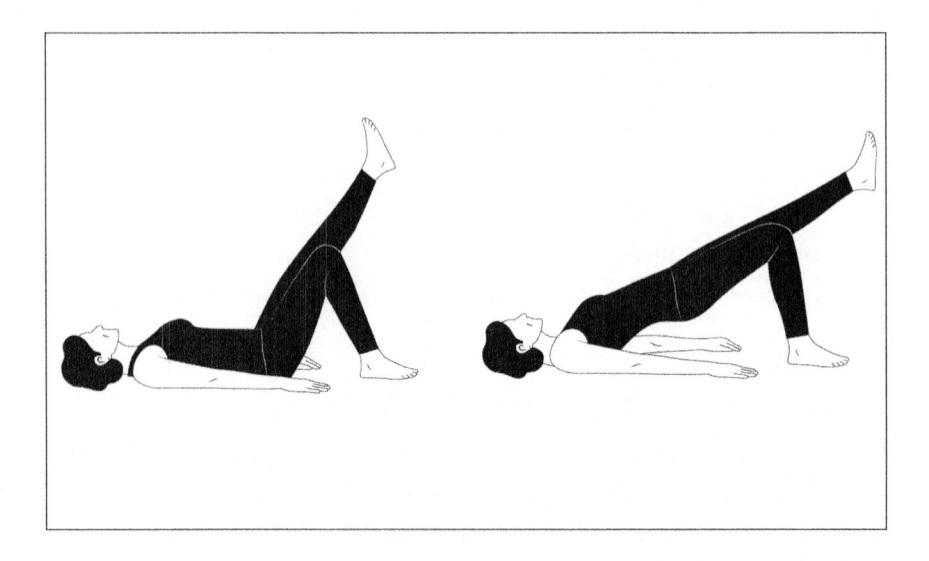

- **Leg Circles:** Lying on your back, bring one leg up and rotate in small circles. Leg circles promote hip joint mobility. The movement range can be adjusted based on individual comfort and flexibility. This activity emphasizes precision and fluidity, enhancing hip mobility while stabilizing the core.

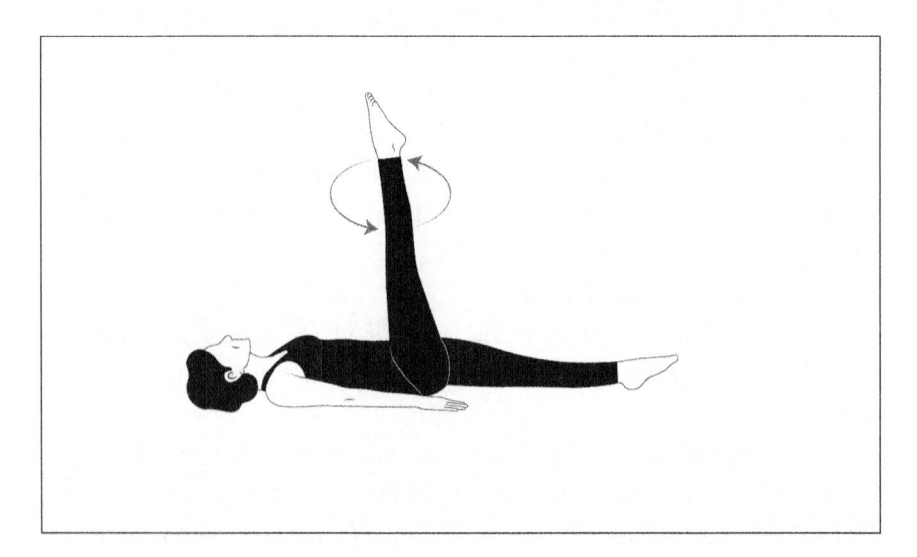

- **Arm Openings:** Lay on your side with both legs bent at a slight angle. With your arms on the same side as your knees are bent, slowly open your arms while keeping your legs together. Allow your head to follow the movement of your arm. This exercise enhances shoulder mobility and opens up the chest, combating the forward hunch that can develop with arthritis in the spine and shoulders.

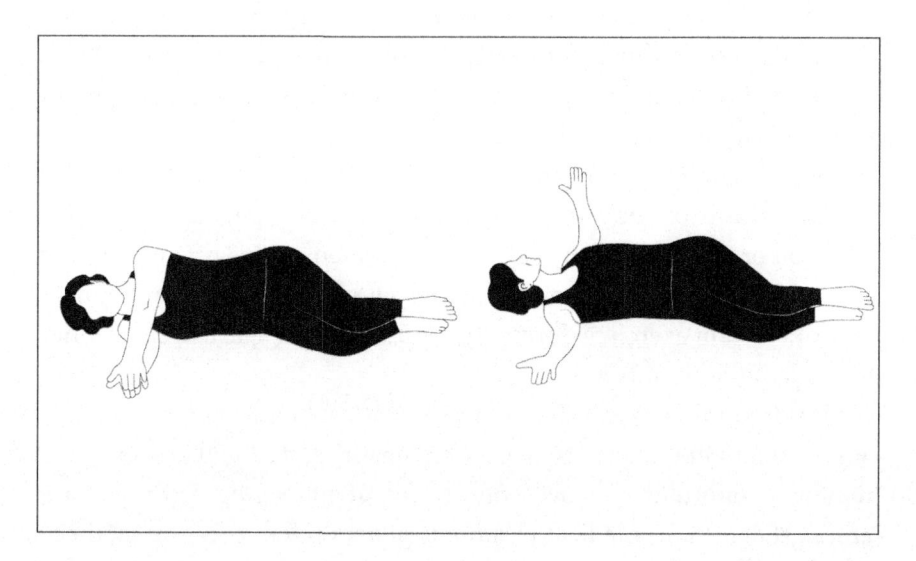

Each exercise targets areas commonly impacted by arthritis, aiming to strengthen surrounding muscles, enhance mobility, and offer relief from stiffness and pain.

Modifications for Arthritis Sufferers

Not all Pilates exercises suit everyone, especially those with arthritis. Modifications ensure that individuals can perform exercises safely and without discomfort:

- **Use of Props:** Props like pillows for support, resistance bands for gentle strengthening, or chairs for seated exercises help in modifying movements to accommodate limited mobility.
- **Reduced Range of Motion:** Limiting the range of motion in exercises like leg circles helps prevent joint overextension, reducing the risk of pain or injury.
- **Alternative Positions:** For some, lying flat might be uncomfortable. Pilates offers the flexibility to perform certain exercises in sitting or standing positions, utilizing the wall for support if necessary.

These modifications are key in making Pilates accessible and beneficial for individuals with arthritis, ensuring that exercises strengthen without exacerbating joint pain.

Integrating Pilates with Medical Treatment Plans

While Pilates offers significant benefits for managing arthritis pain, it is most effective when part of a comprehensive treatment plan. Coordination with healthcare providers is crucial to ensure that Pilates complements medical treatments. This collaborative approach allows for a holistic management plan that addresses arthritis from multiple angles, optimizing health outcomes.

Healthcare providers can offer guidance on specific exercises to focus on or avoid based on an individual's medical history and current condition. For instance, someone with rheumatoid arthritis might need to avoid certain exercises during flare-ups but can engage in them when the inflammation subsides.

Furthermore, healthcare professionals can monitor progress and adjust treatment plans as necessary, ensuring that Pilates exercises remain a safe and effective component of managing arthritis. Integrating Pilates into medical treatment plans underscores the method's value as part of a holistic approach to health and well-being for individuals with arthritis.

Through Pilates, individuals suffering from arthritis can find a powerful ally in their quest for pain relief and improved mobility. The method's low-impact, adaptable nature ensures that exercises can be tailored to meet individual needs, offering a gentle yet effective way to enhance joint health. Modifications and integrating Pilates into broader medical treatment plans further ensure that individuals can practice safely, maximizing the benefits of Pilates for arthritis management. As such, Pilates stands not just as an exercise method but as a comprehensive approach to improving the quality of life for those affected by arthritis.

2.9 PILATES FOR OSTEOPOROSIS: SAFE PRACTICES FOR BONE HEALTH

Osteoporosis is a condition that weakens bones, making them fragile and more likely to break. It's a significant concern for seniors, as it can severely impact mobility and independence. However, not all forms of exercise are created equal regarding osteoporosis. Pilates, with its emphasis on controlled, low-impact movements, stands out as a particularly beneficial practice for those looking to support their bone health safely.

Understanding Osteoporosis and Exercise

The right kind of exercise can play a crucial role in managing osteoporosis. It works in two key ways: by slowing the rate of bone loss and by reducing the risk of falls through improved balance and strength. Pilates, known for its focus on core strength, balance, and flexibility, aligns perfectly with these goals. It encourages movements that stimulate bone strengthening without placing undue stress on the body. However, it's vital to approach Pilates with an awareness of how to modify exercises to avoid putting fragile bones at risk.

Recommended Pilates Exercises for Bone Strengthening

Several Pilates exercises are especially beneficial for individuals with osteoporosis, focusing on building bone density and improving overall stability:

- **Standing Toe Raises:** This simple weight-bearing exercise strengthens the legs and promotes balance. Slowly rising to your toes and lowering back down engages the muscles and bones in the lower legs, encouraging bone growth. The exercise emphasizes controlled, steady elevation and lowering of the heels, targeting the calf muscles and encouraging proprioceptive awareness.

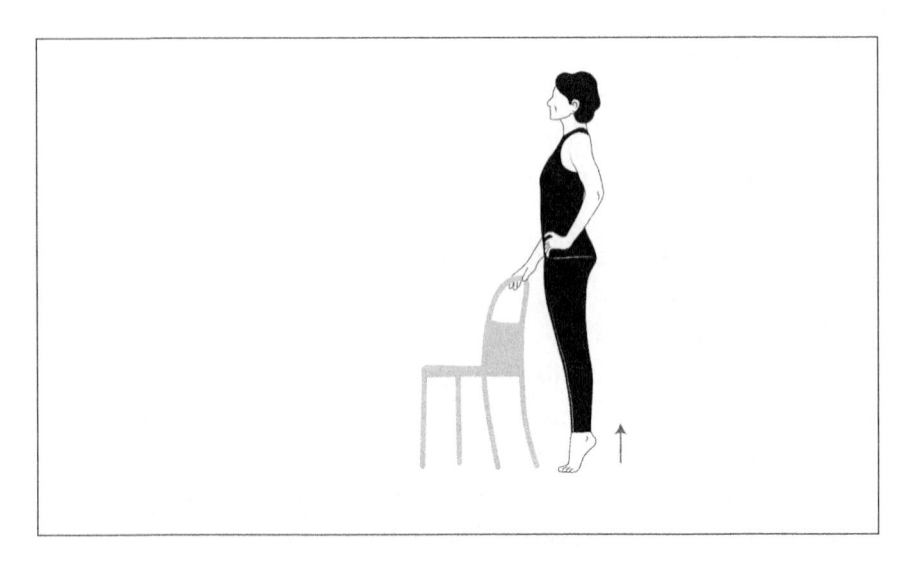

- **Modified Pilates Chair Squats:** Squats are excellent for leg and hip strength but must be changed for osteoporosis patients. Using a chair for support, perform small, controlled squats to engage the thigh and hip muscles without bending deeply. Stand in front of the chair with feet hip-width apart. Slowly lower your body towards the chair as if about to sit, move your hips backward, and keep your knees over your toes. Just before touching the chair, pause and rise back to a standing position. This modified squat focuses on controlled descent and ascent, emphasizing proper posture and muscle engagement without the full weight-bearing impact of a regular squat.

GENTLE WALL PILATES FOR SENIORS:

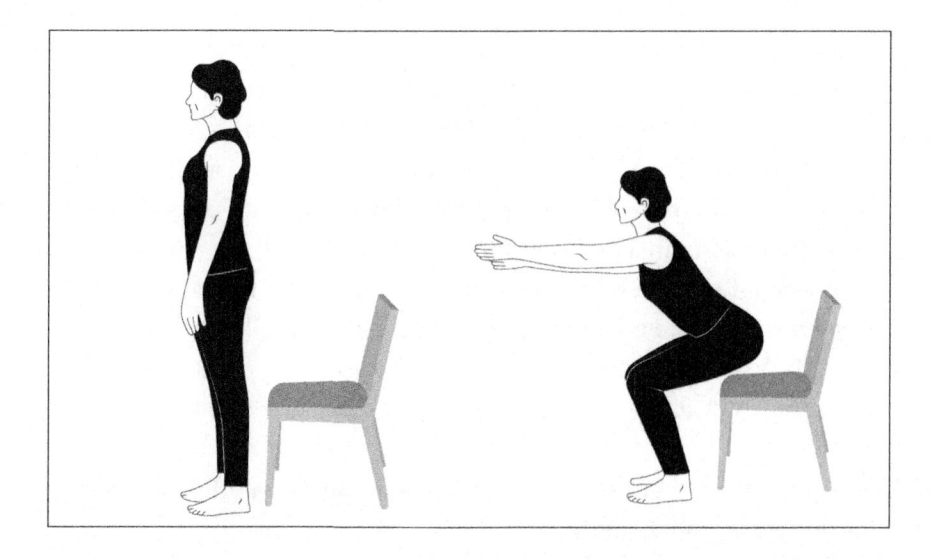

• **Pelvic Curl:** Lying on your back with knees bent, slowly lift your pelvis towards the ceiling, then lower it back down. This movement strengthens the spine and buttocks in a safe, controlled manner. This exercise emphasizes smooth, controlled movement to strengthen the core, glutes, and hamstrings while enhancing spinal mobility.

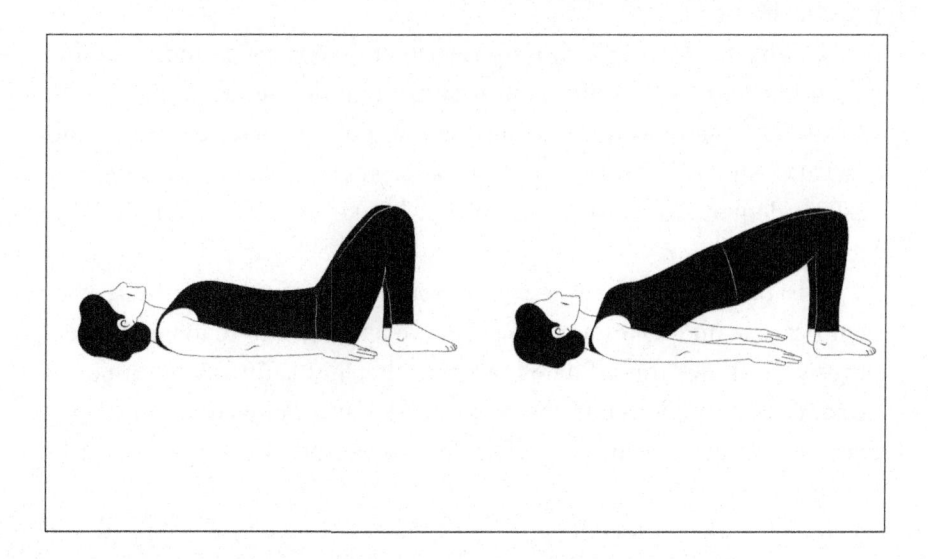

Incorporating these exercises into your Pilates routine can help enhance bone strength and reduce the risk of fractures.

Avoiding High-Risk Movements

When practicing Pilates with osteoporosis, it's crucial to avoid or modify specific movements to prevent injury:

- **Twisting Movements:** Exercises that involve twisting the spine can increase the risk of fractures in weakened bones. Focus on movements that maintain a neutral spine.
- **Deep Bends:** Avoid exercises involving deep forward bends or stretching the spine too far, as these can pressure fragile vertebrae.
- **High-Impact Exercises:** Stick to low-impact Pilates exercises. Avoid jumps or any movements that jar the body, which could lead to fractures.

Being mindful of these modifications ensures a safe Pilates practice that supports bone health.

Collaboration with Health Professionals

Working closely with healthcare professionals is essential for tailoring your Pilates practice to accommodate osteoporosis. Regular check-ups can monitor bone density and overall health, providing valuable feedback on how Pilates contributes to bone health. This collaborative approach ensures your Pilates routine is safe and optimized for your health needs.

Healthcare providers can advise which exercises to focus on and which to avoid based on the latest clinical guidelines and your health history. They can also provide insights into other lifestyle adjustments that may support your Pilates practice, such as dietary changes to ensure adequate calcium and vitamin D intake, which are vital for bone health.

This partnership between you, your Pilates instructor, and your healthcare team creates a comprehensive approach to managing osteoporosis. It allows for a Pilates practice that not only safely enhances bone strength but also enriches your overall well-being, enabling you to maintain an active, fulfilling lifestyle despite the challenges posed by osteoporosis.

2.10 MOBILITY AND INDEPENDENCE: PILATES EXERCISES THAT EMPOWER

Staying active and maintaining independence are vital goals for many seniors. The role of Pilates in achieving these objectives cannot be overstated, particularly when it comes to functional fitness. This form of exercise, characterized by its gentle yet effective movements, helps keep daily activities possible and enjoyable.

Functional fitness refers to the ability to carry out the tasks and activities that are part of our routine life. This could mean anything from carrying groceries to playing with grandchildren for seniors. Focusing on core strength, flexibility, and balance, Pilates directly improves these capabilities. The exercises emphasize movements that are not just beneficial within the confines of a class but extend their advantages to the movements of everyday life.

A set of Pilates exercises specifically designed to enhance mobility focuses on increasing the range of motion and strengthening muscles in a way that mirrors daily activities. For instance:

• **Arm Reaches and Leg Stretches:** Simulating the actions of reaching for items on high shelves or picking things up from the ground, these exercises strengthen the muscles involved in these actions, making them easier and safer to perform.

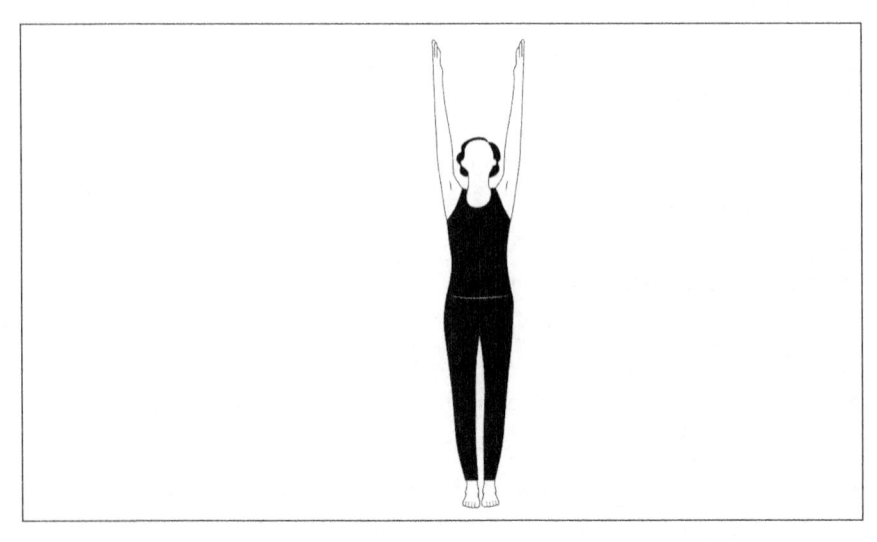

Arm Reaches

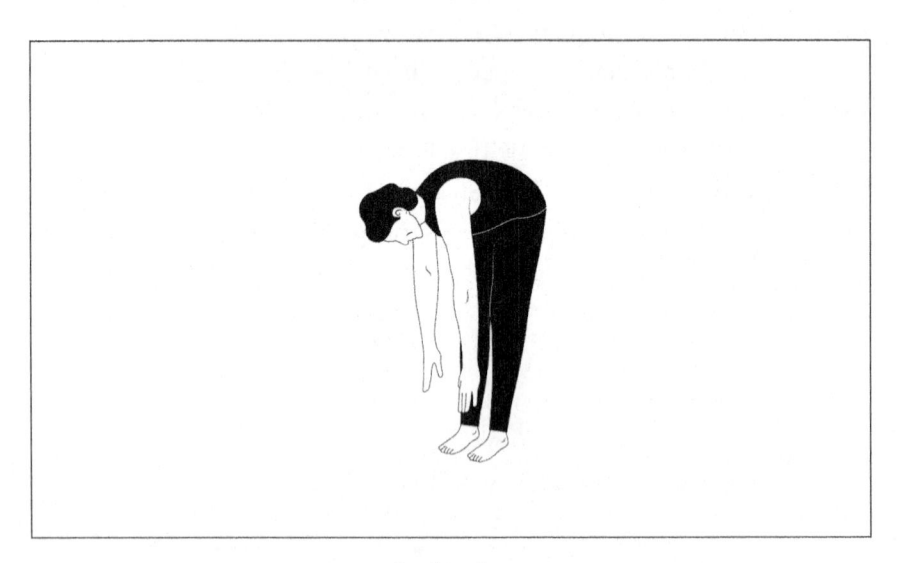

Leg Stretches

- **Chair Stands:** By practicing standing up from a seated position without using hands, seniors can improve their leg strength and balance, which is crucial for maintaining mobility independence. While seated, with your feet flat on the ground, hip-width apart, engage your core, and lean slightly forward. Without using your hands, press through your heels to stand up, extending the hips and knees fully. Carefully lower yourself back to the seated position and repeat.

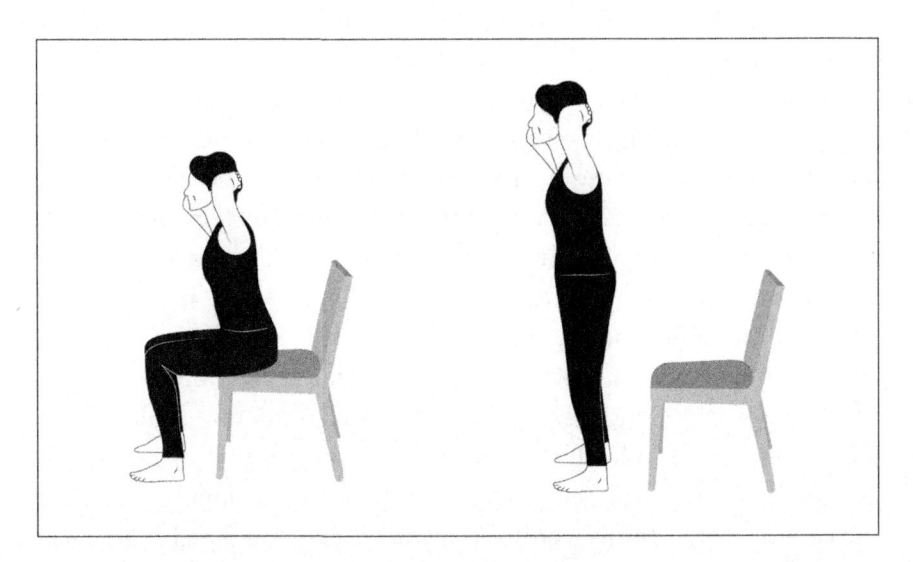

These examples illustrate how Pilates exercises can be directly applied to everyday tasks, enhancing the ease with which they are performed.

The testament to Pilates' effectiveness in promoting independence and mobility comes through in the stories of seniors who have seen significant improvements in their quality of life. One remarkable example is an individual who, after incorporating Pilates into their routine, found they could garden for more extended periods without the back pain that used to cut their hobby short. Another senior regained the confidence to take solo walks in their neighborhood, something they had not felt secure doing for years due to balance concerns.

Customizing Pilates routines to meet individual needs is pivotal in ensuring the exercises are beneficial and enjoyable. This customization might involve adjusting the intensity of the exercises, using props for support, or focusing on specific areas of mobility that an individual wishes to improve. The key lies in tailoring the practice to the person, not vice versa.

. . .

When developing a customized Pilates routine, consider the following:

- **Personal Goals**: Whether improving balance, strengthening the legs, or enhancing overall flexibility, setting clear goals can guide the customization of the Pilates routine.
- **Health Conditions**: Tailoring exercises to work around existing health conditions ensures the practice is safe and beneficial.
- **Preferences**: Incorporating preferred movements or exercises can make the routine more enjoyable, encouraging regular practice.

In wrapping up this exploration of Pilates' role in promoting mobility and independence among seniors, it's clear that this form of exercise is more than just a series of movements. It's a pathway to maintaining an active, independent lifestyle well into our senior years. Pilates empowers individuals to tackle their daily activities confidently and easily through tailored routines focusing on functional fitness. The success stories of those who have regained or maintained their independence through Pilates underscore the transformative potential of this practice.

As we move forward, bear in mind Pilates's overarching empowerment theme. It's not just about the physical benefits but about enhancing the quality of life, enabling seniors to enjoy their daily activities more easily and confidently.

3

DESIGNING A PERSONAL PILATES AREA AT HOME

Imagine transforming a corner of your home into an inviting and serene space that stepping into it lifts your spirits and motivates you to move, breathe, and stretch. This chapter is all about turning that vision into reality. After all, the ambiance of your exercise area can significantly affect your mindset and performance. Whether you have a sprawling living room or a cozy nook, setting up a dedicated Pilates space is simpler than you might think.

Designating a Dedicated Space
- **Why It Matters:** A specific spot for Pilates signals your brain that it's time for self-care and focus. It can be as simple as moving a coffee table to the side or as dedicated as an entire room.
- **Choosing Your Spot:** Look for an area with natural light and enough space to stretch out fully. If you're in a smaller space, consider furniture that's easy to shift around.
- **Making It Yours:** Personalize this space. Maybe it's a photo of a serene landscape or a small plant. These touches make the space inviting, encouraging you to return day after day.

Essential Equipment and Modifications

• **The Basics:** At its core, Pilates requires minimal equipment. A mat and your body weight are enough to get started. However, a few additions can enhance your practice.

▪ **Pilates Mat:** Thicker than a yoga mat, it provides cushioning for your spine during floor exercises.

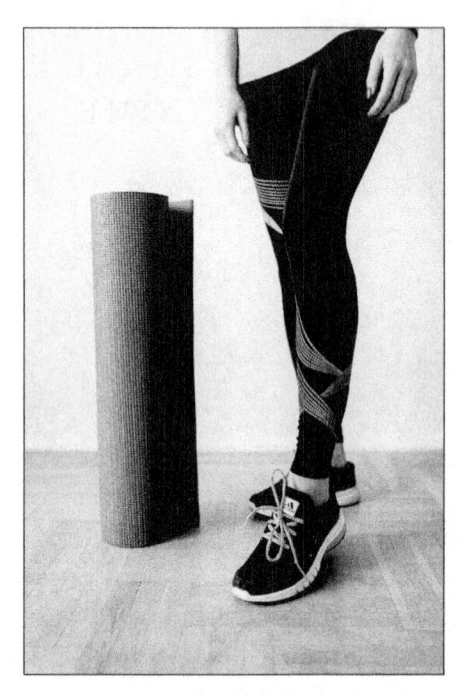

Pilates Mat

▪ **Resistance Bands:** These offer a way to add resistance to exercises without heavy weights, ideal for strengthening and flexibility work.

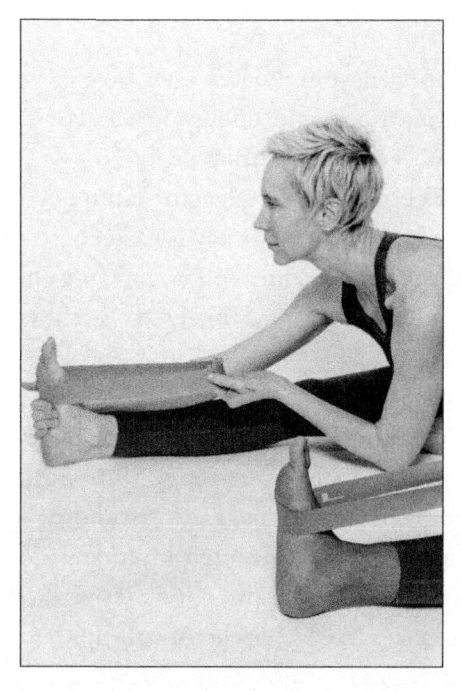

Resistance Bands

- **Magic Circle:** This flexible ring provides resistance for muscle toning, particularly for inner and outer thighs.

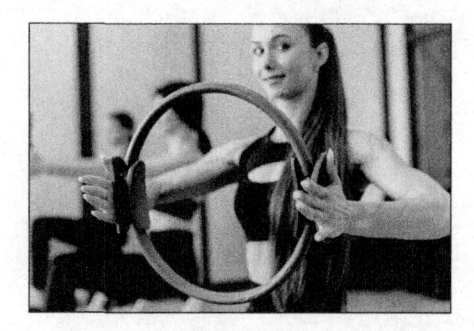

Magic Circle

- **DIY Alternatives:** No Pilates ring? No problem. A sturdy cushion can serve for seated exercises, and a towel can replace a resistance band in a pinch.

. . .

Creating an Inviting Atmosphere

- **Lighting:** Position your Pilates area near a window if you can. Natural light boosts mood and energy levels. For evening sessions, a soft lamp can create a calming ambiance.
- **Declutter:** Keep the space clear of clutter. When your exercise area is tidy, focusing and moving freely is easier.
- **Temperature:** Ensure the room isn't too hot or cold. Being comfortable means you're more likely to stick with your practice without distractions.

Safety Considerations

- **Flooring:** A non-slip surface is crucial. Hardwood floors with a Pilates mat or a carpet that doesn't bunch up are ideal options. This prevents slips and provides stability during standing exercises.
- **Space Clearance:** Ensure enough room around your mat to fully extend your arms and legs in all directions. This freedom of movement is essential for exercises like leg circles or roll-ups.
- **Equipment Storage:** Keep your Pilates gear neatly stored but easily accessible. This way, setting up for your session is quick and hassle-free, making it more likely you'll stick to your routine.

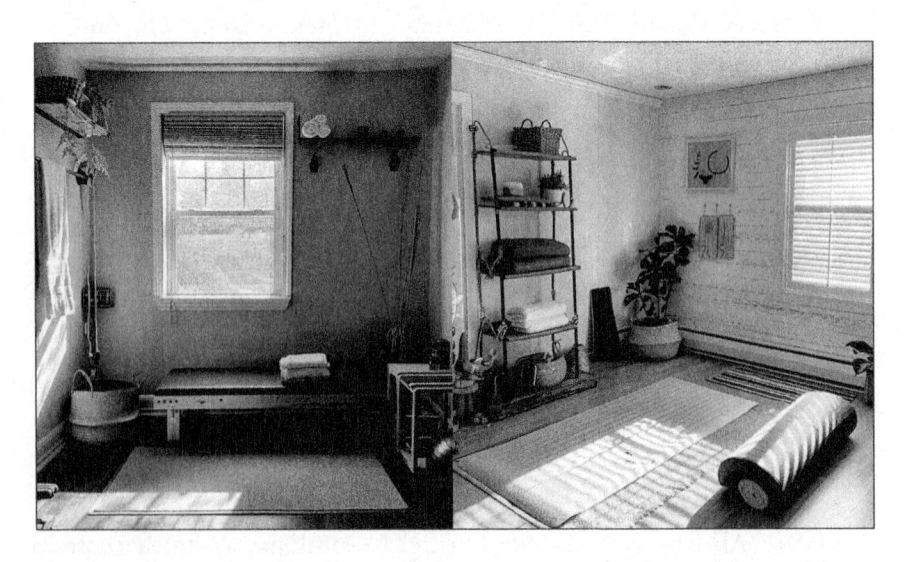

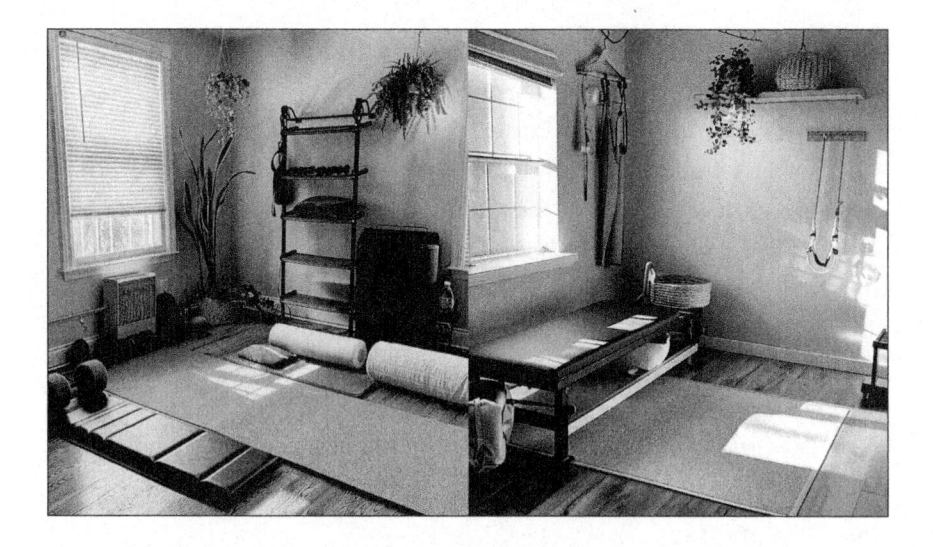

A checklist for setting up your Pilates space could include:
- Pilates mat placed on a non-slip surface
- Resistance bands and Pilates ring stored within arm's reach
- A small shelf or basket for water and a towel
- Space cleared around the mat for unrestricted movement

Creating a dedicated spot for your Pilates practice at home doesn't require a big budget or a lot of space. It's about carving out a little area where you can focus on your health and well-being, free from the distractions of daily life. With some thought and creativity, you can turn even the smallest corner into a Pilates haven that beckons you to take a break from the world and tune into your body's needs. Remember, this space reflects your commitment to yourself, a physical manifestation of your dedication to maintaining mobility, strength, and balance as you age.

3.1 INCORPORATING PILATES INTO YOUR DAILY ROUTINE

Crafting a daily routine that includes Pilates requires creativity, flexibility, and a dash of ingenuity. It's about weaving the practice into the fabric of your day so seamlessly that it feels less like an added task and more like a natural part of your rhythm. Let's explore how you can sprinkle Pilates throughout your day, making it as habitual as your morning coffee or evening wind-down.

Identifying Opportune Times

The key to integrating Pilates into your day is spotting those golden moments that are ripe for movement. Perhaps it's the tranquility of early morning before the household stirs or the calm that follows dinner. Reflect on your daily schedule and pinpoint when a quick session could be most beneficial and least disruptive. It might help to:

• Maintain a log for a few days, jotting down your activities and noting potential slots for Pilates.

• Pay attention to when you feel most energetic versus when you could use a pick-me-up. Aligning your practice with these times maximizes its impact.

Short Sessions for Busy Days

We all have days packed to the brim, where dedicating even half an hour to Pilates seems like a stretch. Remember that a short session is infinitely better than none on such days. Consider these strategies:

• Break your practice into "Pilates moments," five-minute bursts of activity you can do between tasks. A series of standing leg lifts while waiting for the coffee to brew or a quick spine stretch before hopping into the shower can invigorate and refresh.

• Have a set of go-to movements that require minimal setup. This way, you can jump right into a quick session without hesitation.

Making Pilates a Habit

The transformation of Pilates from an occasional activity to a daily habit hinges on your approach. Here are a few strategies to embed Pilates into the very essence of your everyday life:

• Anchor your Pilates practice to an existing habit. Tagging a few Pilates stretches onto your morning routine can help cement it as part of your start-the-day ritual.

• Set gentle reminders around your home. A Pilates mat left invitingly open, a sticky note on the bathroom mirror, or setting an alarm can serve as prompts to practice.

Family and Household Involvement

Pilates can transcend personal practice, becoming a conduit for connection and shared experiences within the household. Engaging those you live with in your practice fosters support and can turn it into a fun, joint activity. Here's how you might involve them:

• Invite them to join you for a session. A partner or family Pilates session can be an excellent way to spend quality time together while staying active.

• Turn Pilates into a game with children or grandchildren. Who can hold a pose the longest or has the most graceful roll-up? This not only makes it enjoyable for them but also keeps you motivated.

In weaving Pilates into the fabric of your daily life, the aim is to shift from viewing it as a discrete task to embracing it as an integral part of your lifestyle. This shift doesn't happen overnight but evolves through mindful scheduling, abbreviated sessions to accommodate busier days, customary practice, and involving those around you for support and camaraderie. Pilates becomes more than just an exercise—it becomes a daily touchstone for balance, strength, and serenity.

3.2 SHORT AND SWEET: THE 10-MINUTE PILATES WORKOUT FOR BUSY DAYS

In the realm of Pilates, there's a golden nugget of wisdom that advocates for the power of brevity in practice. These are the micro-workouts tailored explicitly for those days when time is a luxury you can't afford. The beauty of these 10-minute routines lies in their simplicity and effectiveness, proving that even in a brief window, you can invigorate your body, sharpen your mind, and uplift your spirit.

Effective Micro-Workouts

Introducing the concept of micro-workouts opens up a world where every minute counts. These compact routines are designed to pack a punch, targeting key areas of the body to ensure a comprehensive workout, even on time-crunched days. Here's how you can dive into a 10-minute session:

• Start with a two-minute warm-up, focusing on deep, thoracic breathing to awaken your senses and prep your muscles.

• Follow up with a series of mat exercises, dedicating one minute to each movement. Think pelvic curls, spine stretches, and single-leg circles that engage your core, stretch your spine and mobilize your hips.

- Conclude with a two-minute cool-down, returning to your breath, allowing for a gentle transition back into your day.

Routine Variations

To keep your Pilates practice fresh and challenging, rotating through different 10-minute routines is essential. This strategy prevents monotony and ensures a balanced approach, targeting various muscle groups throughout the week. Consider these variations:

- **Core Focus:** Center your session around abdominal and lower back exercises, reinforcing your core's stability and strength.
- **Legs and Glutes:** Allocate your minutes to exercises that tone your lower body, building endurance and power in your legs and buttocks.
- **Upper Body and Arms:** Shift your attention to movements that strengthen your shoulders, chest, and arms, using your body weight or resistance bands for added challenge.

Diversifying your routines keeps your muscles guessing and your mind engaged, fostering physical and mental agility.

The Power of Consistency

The magic ingredient in these micro-workouts is consistency. While each session might seem like a drop in the ocean, these drops create ripples, significantly improving strength, flexibility, and mental well-being over time. Consistency transforms these brief Pilates segments into a powerful tool for health maintenance, proving that it's not the duration but the regularity of your practice that counts. Here's how to stay on track:

- Schedule your Pilates time as you would any other important appointment, making it non-negotiable.
- Keep your Pilates mat rolled out or visible as a physical reminder of your commitment to your practice and well-being.
- Celebrate your consistency with small rewards, reinforcing the positive habit you're building.

Incorporating Mindfulness

To amplify the benefits of your 10-minute Pilates workouts, weaving mindfulness into each session turns a simple routine into a holistic practice. Here's how to infuse mindfulness into your movements:

- Before beginning, take a moment to center yourself, setting an intention for your session. This could be as simple as seeking calm or as specific as focusing on fluidity in your movements.

• During exercises, maintain a keen awareness of your breath, allowing it to guide and deepen your movements. This focus enhances the physical benefits of each exercise and calms the mind, creating a meditative quality in your workout.

• Use the final minutes of your session for reflection. Acknowledge your work, thank yourself for the effort, and carry that sense of accomplishment and serenity with you for the rest of your day.

These 10-minute Pilates sessions testify to the idea that quality trumps quantity. By prioritizing effectiveness, variety, consistency, and mindfulness, you ensure that even on the busiest days, you're taking meaningful steps toward your health and wellness goals. This approach demystifies the notion that substantial time investments are necessary for meaningful exercise, offering a practical, flexible solution to staying active and centered, no matter what life throws your way.

3.3 FROM MORNING TO NIGHT: PILATES THROUGHOUT THE DAY

Waking up to a new day offers a blank canvas to paint our wellness routine, and what better way to fill it than with Pilates? This versatile practice can adapt to every part of our day, energizing us in the morning, reinvigorating us during the day, and soothing us into the night. Let's explore how to weave Pilates into the fabric of our daily lives, ensuring we stay limber, strong, and serene from dawn until dusk.

Morning Awakening Routines

The first light of day brings a unique energy, an ideal backdrop for invigorating our body and setting a positive tone for the hours ahead. Morning Pilates routines can be designed to gently wake the body, focusing on exercises that warm the muscles, lubricate the joints, and kickstart our metabolism.

• **Sun Salutations, Pilates Style:** Borrowing from yoga, a modified Sun Salutation sequence can awaken the body. Start with a series of arm raises, moving into a gentle forward bend, followed by a careful step back into a plank, and concluding with a downward dog stretch.

Each movement is synchronized with our breath, drawing energy in with every inhale and releasing tension with every exhale.

- **Dynamic Leg Swings:** Holding onto a chair or wall for support, gently swing one leg forward and back, then switch to the other leg. This not only warms up the hip joints but also stimulates blood circulation.

Midday Movement Breaks

As the day progresses, our energy can wane, particularly if we've been stationary for extended periods. Integrating Pilates into our midday routine can counteract the effects of prolonged sitting, re-energize our minds, and refresh our focus.

- **Chair-assisted Pilates:** While seated, simple Pilates exercises like seated leg lifts or spine twists can invigorate the body without needing to change into workout gear. These movements bring our attention back to our core, encouraging us to sit taller and breathe more deeply.
- **Standing Stretch and Balance:** Taking a break to stand, we can engage in a series of standing stretches, like reaching high with both arms and bending gently to each side. Balancing on one foot, then the other, for a count of ten, helps reactivate our sense of balance and coordination, which is crucial for maintaining muscle tone and bone health.

Evening Wind-Down Exercises

As evening falls, our focus shifts towards unwinding and preparing our body for rest. Pilates routines at this time should emphasize relaxation, stretching, and releasing the day's tensions, promoting a night of deep and restorative sleep.

- **Gentle Mat Work:** Exercises performed on the mat, such as the pelvic curl or a slow-paced hundred, can help decompress the spine and relax the muscles. Incorporating props like a small pillow under the head or a blanket can enhance comfort, making the transition to relaxation smoother.

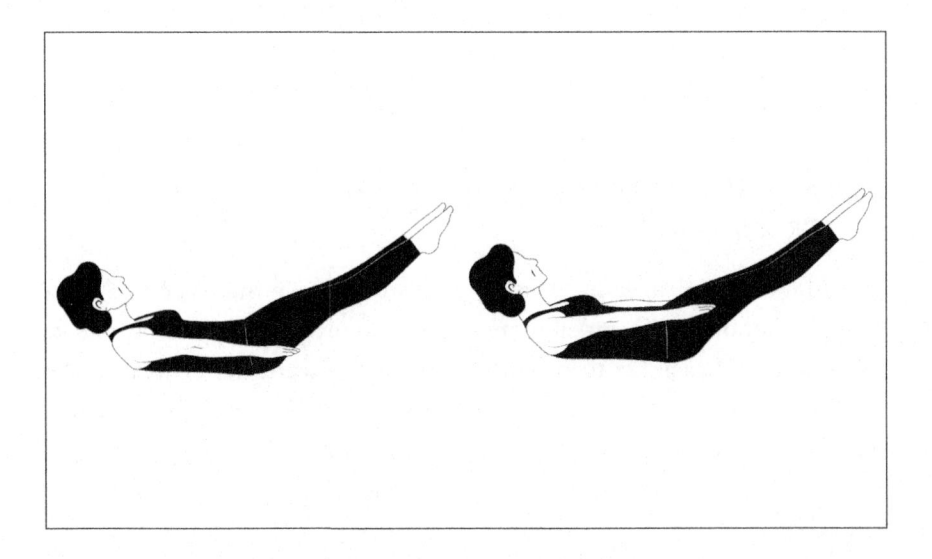

- **Breathing for Relaxation:** Ending the day with focused breathing exercises helps calm the nervous system. Lying on the back with hands resting on the abdomen, deep diaphragmatic breaths help release physical and mental tension, preparing us for a peaceful sleep.

Adapting Routines to Energy Levels

Our energy levels ebb and flow, influenced by many factors, from sleep quality to daily stressors. Adapting our Pilates practice to match our energy levels ensures we always nurture our body, never draining it.

- **Listen to Your Body:** Some days, we feel capable of a more vigorous routine, while others call for gentleness. Tuning into our body's signals allows us to choose exercises that match our needs, ensuring Pilates remains a source of rejuvenation rather than exhaustion.
- **Modifying Exercises:** On days when energy is low, modifying exercises to be performed sitting or even lying down can help maintain our practice without overexertion. Conversely, adding small weights or increasing repetitions can amplify the challenge when energy abounds.

Incorporating Pilates from morning to night offers a holistic approach to wellness, ensuring we have the tools to remain balanced, strong, and serene no matter what the day brings. By listening to our bodies and adapting our routines, we ensure Pilates remains a faithful companion, supporting us through every phase of our day and every stage of our lives.

3.4 ENGAGING WITH TECHNOLOGY: USING APPS FOR PROGRESS TRACKING

In today's digital age, harnessing technology to enhance our Pilates practice not only adds an element of convenience but also empowers us with data and insights to refine our journey toward better health. For seniors, navigating through a sea of apps might initially seem daunting. Yet, finding the right tools can transform your Pilates regimen from a solitary pursuit into an engaging, trackable, and socially connected experience.

Selecting the Right Apps

Diving into the world of Pilates and fitness apps opens up many choices. Here's what to look for to ensure the app you choose is a perfect fit for your senior Pilates practice:

- **User-Friendliness:** Opt for apps with intuitive interfaces. Large text, clear instructions, and easy navigation are key factors that cater to all users, regardless of their tech savvy.
- **Customization Options:** Everyone's fitness journey is unique. An app that can tailor routines to your needs, limitations, and goals will be most beneficial.
- **Progress Tracking Features:** Look for apps that offer detailed tracking of your workouts, progress over time, and even reminders for your next session. This functionality can be instrumental in keeping you motivated.
- **Community and Support:** Some apps provide access to online communities. This can be a great source of encouragement, sharing experiences, and getting advice from fellow Pilates enthusiasts.

Benefits of Digital Tracking

Incorporating technology for progress tracking in your Pilates practice comes with several advantages:

- **Motivation Boost:** Seeing tangible progress over time can significantly boost your motivation. It's rewarding to look back and see how far you've come.

- **Consistency**: Apps that send workout reminders can help you maintain regularity in your practice. Consistency is critical to reaping the full benefits of Pilates.
- **Personalized Feedback**: Some apps analyze your progress and offer feedback or suggestions for improvement. This can help you adjust your practice for better results.

Privacy and Safety

While technology offers numerous benefits, it's crucial to navigate it with an awareness of privacy and security, especially when health data is involved:

- **Read Privacy Policies**: Before downloading an app, take the time to understand how your data will be used and stored. Look for apps that prioritize user privacy.
- **Use Secure Networks**: When using fitness apps, ensure your internet connection is secure, especially if entering personal information.
- **Be Selective with Shared Information**: Only share what's necessary. Be cautious about entering sensitive health data unless it's essential for the app's functionality.

Alternatives to Digital Tracking

For those who prefer a more traditional or less tech-centric approach, there are effective ways to track your Pilates progress:

- **Pilates Journals**: Keeping a physical journal where you log your routines, feelings, and observations can be a deeply personal way to track progress. Reflecting on your entries can offer insights and motivation similar to digital apps.
- **Printed Charts**: Simple charts with exercises listed for each day of the week can help you plan and track your Pilates workouts. Marking off completed sessions can visually represent your consistency and dedication.
- **Buddy System**: Partnering with a friend or family member to share your Pilates goals and achievements can offer a blend of accountability and support. Regular check-ins can serve as a reminder and motivation to keep progressing.

In an era where technology intersects with almost every aspect of our lives, knowing we have tools at our fingertips to enhance our Pilates practice is empowering. Whether you embrace app technology for its tracking capabilities and convenience or opt for more traditional methods, the key is to find a system that works for you and keeps you engaged, informed, and motivated on your path to better health and well-being through Pilates.

3.5 THE POWER OF HABIT: MAKING PILATES A DAILY RITUAL

Making Pilates an inseparable part of your day, akin to morning coffee or evening strolls, requires more than just a sprinkle of willpower. It calls for a strategic approach to habit formation, an understanding of the power of consistency, and a toolbox for overcoming the hurdles that life might throw your way. Let's unwrap these layers, one by one, to see how Pilates can seamlessly weave itself into the fabric of your daily life.

Habit Formation Strategies

The science of habit formation tells us that the path to embedding a new practice like Pilates into our lives isn't just about repetition but about creating a structure that supports this repetition. Here's how:

- Start Small: Begin with manageable Pilates sessions that don't overwhelm you. A commitment to even five minutes a day is better than none.
- Attach It to an Existing Habit: Link your Pilates practice to another well-established part of your routine. After brushing your teeth, for example, roll out your mat.
- Be Specific: Rather than a vague "I'll do Pilates today," plan exactly when and where you'll practice. "I'll do Pilates in the living room at 7:30 AM," sets a clear action plan.

Role of Consistency

The cornerstone of making Pilates a habit lies in consistency rather than intensity. The regularity of your practice, not how long or hard you work out, builds and solidifies this new habit. Consistency:

- Trains Your Brain: Regular practice helps your brain to encode Pilates as a default behavior, something you do without having to debate or decide.
- Builds Momentum: Each consecutive day you practice, you're

building strength, flexibility, and mental and emotional resilience toward making Pilates a non-negotiable part of your day.

Cue-Routine-Reward Cycle

Diving deeper into habit formation, the Cue-Routine-Reward cycle emerges as a robust framework. Here's how it applies to Pilates:

- **Cue:** Identify a consistent trigger reminding you it's time for Pilates. This could be a visual cue, like seeing your Pilates mat out, or a temporal cue, such as a specific time of day.
- **Routine:** This is your Pilates practice. The key is to make this as seamless and enjoyable as possible. Having your equipment ready and choosing routines you enjoy can make a big difference.
- **Reward:** Reward yourself after each Pilates session. This doesn't have to be elaborate; it could be a moment of relaxation, a favorite healthy treat, or simply marking off the session on your calendar. This reward helps to reinforce the habit loop.

Overcoming Common Barriers

As with any habit, there will be days when motivation wanes or time seems like a scarce commodity. Here are strategies to navigate these barriers:

- Lack of Time: Break down your practice into smaller, more manageable segments. Remember, a few minutes of Pilates is better than none. Utilize those short bursts of time you might otherwise spend scrolling through your phone.
- Waning Motivation: Keep a motivation journal to jot down how you feel after each Pilates session. Reading through this on more challenging days can be a powerful motivator. Additionally, vary your routines to keep things exciting and engaging.
- Feeling Overwhelmed: If the thought of an entire session feels daunting, permit yourself to do less. Acknowledge that any practice is a success.

In weaving Pilates into the daily tapestry of our lives, we're not merely adopting a new exercise routine; we're nurturing a practice that enhances our physical well-being, elevates our mood, and anchors our day in mindfulness and intention. This journey of making Pilates a daily ritual is punctuated not by the challenges we might face but by the strategies we employ to overcome them, ensuring that Pilates becomes as much a part of our daily rhythm as the sunrise and sunset.

3.6 PILATES AND SOCIALIZATION: FORMING YOUR SUPPORT GROUP

In the tapestry of wellness, the threads of social connections hold a special significance, especially as we age. It's not just about staying physically active but nurturing those bonds that enrich our lives. Pilates offers a unique avenue for this, blending the benefits of physical exercise with the joy of social interaction. Whether you're reaching out to form a new Pilates circle or joining an existing one, the camaraderie found in these groups can be a source of motivation, support, and joy.

Building a Pilates Community

The path to forming or finding a Pilates community might start at your doorstep or on your digital devices. Here are ways to connect:

- **Local Community Centers and Gyms**: These are often hubs for Pilates classes catering to different skill levels, including seniors. Joining these classes can introduce you to fellow Pilates enthusiasts.
- **Online Platforms**: Social media groups and online forums dedicated to Pilates offer spaces to discuss, learn, and even participate in virtual sessions. These platforms can connect you with a global Pilates community.

The benefits of being part of a Pilates community extend beyond the mat. Sharing the journey enhances motivation, provides a network of support, and enriches the Pilates experience with diverse perspectives.

Group Practice Sessions

Practicing Pilates in a group, whether in-person or virtually, adds a layer of accountability and encouragement. Consider these ideas for group sessions:

- **Host a Pilates Party**: Invite friends or neighbors for a Pilates session in your home or a local park. A group setting can make the practice more enjoyable and less intimidating for beginners.
- **Virtual Pilates Meet-ups**: For those who prefer or require the convenience of home practice, organizing virtual meet-ups through

video calls can keep the sense of community alive. It allows for flexibility in scheduling and the comfort of practicing in your own space.

Group sessions' shared energy and collective focus can elevate your Pilates practice, making each session something to look forward to.

Sharing Progress and Tips

Every member's journey is a source of inspiration and learning within a Pilates community. Engaging in meaningful exchanges about progress, challenges, and insights can foster a deeper connection to the practice. Here's how:

- **Success Stories:** Share your milestones, no matter how small they may seem. Your achievement could be the motivation someone else needs.
- **Exchange Tips:** Found a way to perfect a challenging pose? Discovered a helpful modification? Sharing these tips can help others in their practice.
- **Feedback Sessions:** Constructive feedback can be invaluable. These exchanges can propel everyone forward, whether it's advice on improving form or suggestions for overcoming plateaus.

This culture of sharing not only strengthens the community bond but also accelerates collective growth and improvement.

Social Accountability

One of the most powerful aspects of a Pilates community is the accountability it brings to your practice. Knowing that others count on your presence and participation can be a strong motivator. Here are ways to harness this:

- **Commit to Regular Sessions:** Set a regular schedule for group Pilates sessions. Consistency strengthens the habits of everyone involved.
- **Check-ins:** Regular check-ins with your Pilates friends can keep you accountable. A simple message asking if they've done their Pilates today or sharing that you've completed your session can inspire action.
- **Challenge Each Other:** Set group challenges, such as a daily Pilates streak for a month or mastering a particular set of exercises. Challenges can add an element of fun and competition that keeps everyone engaged.

The accountability factor in a social setting ensures regularity in your Pilates practice and deepens the commitment to your health and wellness goals.

In weaving the threads of socialization into your Pilates practice, you're not just building a support network but enriching your whole experience. The joy of shared achievement, the motivation from being part of a collective, and the accountability that keeps you on track are invaluable. This communal aspect of Pilates adds a vibrant layer to your fitness journey, making it about more than just physical health—it becomes a journey of connection, support, and shared growth.

3.7 STAYING MOTIVATED: CELEBRATING MILESTONES AND PROGRESS

In the realm of Pilates for seniors, motivation acts as the wind beneath the wings of our practice. It's the gentle nudge on days filled with inertia and the congratulatory pat on the back after each session. But how do we keep this motivation aflame, ensuring it doesn't fade? The key lies in setting realistic goals, tracking and celebrating our progress, and understanding what drives us. Let's unravel these threads one by one.

Setting Achievable Goals

The first step towards sustained motivation is to set goals that are within reach. These objectives act as lighthouses, guiding our Pilates voyage through calm and stormy days. Here's how to plot these beacons:

- Start with Clarity: Define what you wish to achieve with your Pilates practice. It could range from improving flexibility to mastering a specific pose. The more precise the goal, the easier it is to navigate.
- Break It Down: Large goals can seem daunting. Break them into smaller, manageable milestones. If you aim to enhance flexibility, your initial milestone could be to perform a full roll-up without assistance.
- Flexibility in Goals: As paradoxical as it might sound, your goals must be flexible. Life throws curveballs, and our bodies respond differently over time. Be prepared to tweak your goals as you progress.

Tracking and Celebrating Progress

Once your goals are set, keeping an eye on the journey toward them becomes crucial. Here's where tracking comes into play, turning abstract goals into tangible achievements.

• Simple Tracking Methods: Use a diary or a calendar to note your daily Pilates activities and any milestones reached. This acts as a visual reminder of how far you've come.

• Celebrate Every Win: Every milestone deserves celebration, no matter how small. Completed a whole week of Pilates without skipping a day? Treat yourself to a relaxing bath or a favorite treat. These celebrations reinforce positive behavior, making you more likely to stick with your routine.

• Share Your Success: Sharing your progress with friends, family, or a Pilates group can multiply the joy. It not only serves as a personal celebration but also inspires others.

Revisiting and Adjusting Goals

The path of Pilates is non-linear, filled with advances and retreats. This necessitates a periodic review and adjustment of your goals.

• Scheduled Reviews: Set aside time monthly or quarterly to review your progress. This could involve reassessing your goals, celebrating achievements, and setting new targets.

• Adaptation Is Key: If certain goals have become too easy or challenging, adjust them. The aim is to align your Pilates practice with your current abilities and aspirations.

Intrinsic vs. Extrinsic Motivation

Understanding what motivates us to roll out our Pilates mat daily can be enlightening. Motivation can be extrinsic, driven by external rewards, or intrinsic, fueled by personal satisfaction.

• Extrinsic Motivators: These could include rewards you give yourself for reaching milestones, encouragement from your Pilates instructor, or the desire to keep up with your Pilates group. While powerful, extrinsic motivators can sometimes wane.

• Intrinsic Motivators: This form of motivation springs from within, such as the joy of movement, the peace that follows a Pilates session, or the satisfaction of improving flexibility. Intrinsic motivators tend to be more enduring.

Balancing these motivators can create a well-rounded approach to maintaining motivation. While rewarding yourself for reaching a goal is wonderful, finding joy in the practice can provide a deeper, more lasting drive to continue.

In the dance of Pilates, staying motivated is akin to keeping the rhythm. It involves setting goals that light up our path, celebrating each step forward, reassessing our direction when needed, and understanding the melody that moves us. This approach ensures that our Pilates practice remains a source of joy, growth, and fulfillment, enriching our lives with every breath and movement.

3.8 ADAPTING YOUR PILATES PRACTICE AS YOU AGE

Our bodies and minds evolve with time, bringing to the fore new strengths and unveiling areas that require extra care. With its inherent adaptability, Pilates can morph alongside us, offering support, strength, and solace through each aging phase. This section delves into how we can fine-tune our Pilates practice, ensuring it remains a steadfast companion that respects our body's changing needs.

Anticipating Changes

Aging is a natural process that introduces various physical and mental adjustments. Our joints might become stiffer, muscles may take longer to warm up, and our concentration could waver more easily than before. Recognizing and anticipating these changes is the first step in adapting our Pilates routine. It's about being proactive rather than reactive, adjusting our practice to preemptively address these shifts. This foresight allows us to continue Pilates safely, minimizing the risk of injury and maximizing the benefits for our well-being.

- **Flexibility Adjustments:** As flexibility wanes, incorporating more dynamic stretches can gently increase our range of motion.
- **Strength Modifications:** Recognizing that muscle strength might not be what it once was, we can introduce props like resistance bands to build strength without overburdening our bodies.
- **Mindfulness Practices:** Incorporating mindfulness and focusing techniques at the beginning of each session can help counterbalance any decrease in concentration, enriching our practice with a more profound sense of presence.

Modifications for Increased Limitations

Adapting exercises to suit our current level of mobility and health is crucial in maintaining a productive and safe Pilates practice. It's about customizing movements to ensure they're achievable, focusing on what we can do rather than what we can't.

- **For Reduced Mobility**: Utilizing chairs for seated exercises or performing movements against a wall can provide stability and support, making exercises more accessible.
- **In Case of Pain or Discomfort**: Substituting exercises that cause discomfort with alternative movements that target the same muscle groups ensures continuity in strengthening without aggravating any conditions.
- **Adjusting Intensity**: Scaling back the intensity of workouts on days when energy levels are low can help maintain a regular practice, honoring our body's signals without pushing beyond comfortable limits.

Enlisting the guidance of a professional, be it a Pilates instructor specializing in senior fitness or a healthcare provider, can offer invaluable insights into tailoring our practice. These experts can help identify the most beneficial modifications, ensuring our Pilates routine supports our health without compromise.

- **Professional Insight**: A Pilates instructor can assess our form and suggest adjustments to enhance the efficacy of each movement, ensuring exercises are performed safely.
- **Healthcare Provider Consultation**: For those navigating specific health conditions, a healthcare provider can offer advice on which Pilates exercises to embrace and which to avoid, aligning our practice with our health needs.

Maintaining a Positive Outlook

Adopting a positive, adaptive outlook towards our evolving Pilates practice is the most crucial adjustment we can make. It's about embracing change with grace, viewing each modification not as a setback but as an evolution of our practice. This mindset shift allows us to appreciate the journey, celebrating the capability and resilience of our bodies at every age.

- **Focus on Achievements**: Celebrating the movements we can perform and the strength we build fosters a sense of achievement and progress, fueling our motivation.

• **Embrace Adaptability**: Viewing each modification as a testament to our commitment to well-being encourages a flexible approach to Pilates that evolves with us.

• **Cultivate Gratitude**: Practicing gratitude for the ability to engage in Pilates, regardless of how our practice looks, deepens our connection to the exercise, transforming it into a source of joy and contentment.

As we move forward, let us remember that Pilates is not just a series of exercises; it's a practice that mirrors life's fluidity, flexing and bending as we do. By anticipating changes, modifying our routines, seeking expert advice, and fostering a positive outlook, we ensure that Pilates remains a nourishing, supportive element of our lives. It becomes a reflection of our resilience, a celebration of our capability, and a testament to our commitment to nurturing our bodies and spirits with kindness and respect.

3.9 PILATES FOR THE MIND: COMBINING MEDITATION AND MOVEMENT

When Pilates and meditation merge, the result is a holistic practice that nurtures both mind and body, creating a synergy that transcends the benefits of each practice alone. This integration offers a pathway to enhanced mental and physical health, providing a balanced approach to wellness that is particularly beneficial as we age.

Integrating Meditation with Pilates

The fusion of Pilates and meditation brings forth a practice where movement and mindfulness coalesce. This fusion amplifies Pilates's physical benefits and introduces a profound layer of mental clarity and tranquility. Here's how you can blend these practices:

• Begin each Pilates session with a few minutes of seated meditation, setting an intention for your practice.

• Use the rhythmic movements of Pilates to anchor your attention in the present moment, turning each exercise into a meditative act.

The advantages of this integrated approach encompass improved focus, reduced stress levels, and a heightened sense of inner peace, making it a powerful tool for enhancing overall well-being.

Mindful Movement

Practicing Pilates with mindfulness means engaging fully with each movement, breath, and moment. This deep engagement brings a quality of attentiveness to our practice, enriching the connection between mind and body. Here are some steps to infuse your Pilates practice with mindfulness:

- As you move through each Pilates exercise, direct your focus to the sensations within your body, observing without judgment.
- Acknowledge the thoughts and emotions that arise during your practice, gently guiding your attention back to your movements and breath.

This mindful approach to Pilates fosters a deeper awareness of our bodies, promotes mental clarity, and enhances the practice's calming effects.

Breathwork as a Bridge

Breathwork in Pilates supports physical movements and serves as a bridge to meditation, deepening the mind-body connection. The conscious control of breathing central to Pilates exercises can be a meditative practice. Techniques to deepen this aspect include:

- Pay close attention to your breath's rhythm and depth as you execute each Pilates movement, using the breath to guide and amplify your exercises.
- Incorporating specific breathing exercises, such as diaphragmatic breathing, before and after your Pilates routine to enhance relaxation and focus.

This focus on breathwork enriches the meditative quality of Pilates, promoting relaxation and mental clarity.

Routines for Mental Wellness

Certain Pilates routines promote mental wellness, reduce stress, and improve cognitive function. These routines often emphasize slow, deliberate movements and deep, mindful breathing. Consider incorporating the following into your practice:

- **The Saw:** This exercise, focusing on controlled movement and breath, can aid in releasing tension and fostering mental calm.

- **Leg Stretches:** Slow leg stretches, combined with focused breathing, can help quiet the mind and reduce anxiety.
- **Spine Twists:** Gentle spine twists encourage mental and physical release, promoting relaxation and mental clarity.

By choosing routines that emphasize the meditative aspects of Pilates, you can enhance your mental wellness, making your practice peaceful for both body and mind.

In weaving meditation into our Pilates practice, we open ourselves to a world where movement heals the body and mind. This holistic approach, emphasizing mindful movement and breath as a bridge to meditation, creates a profoundly nurturing and stimulating practice. The selected routines for mental wellness serve as tools for managing stress, enhancing cognitive function, and promoting a sense of inner peace.

As we close this exploration of Pilates as a holistic practice, we're reminded of the profound interconnectedness of our physical and mental well-being. Through the mindful integration of movement and meditation, Pilates emerges as a form of exercise and a path to a more balanced, serene, and enriched life. As we advance, let's carry forward the understanding that our wellness journey is multifaceted, with each aspect of our practice contributing to the greater tapestry of our health and happiness.

MAKE A DIFFERENCE WITH YOUR REVIEW

"Kindness is the language which the deaf can hear, and the blind can see." - Mark Twain.

Hello, wonderful people!

Did you know those who do kind things for others might have the happiest hearts? And if there's a chance we can do that right here and now, you bet we're going to take it!

So, here's something I'm really curious about...

Would you be willing to lend a hand to someone you've never met, even if you didn't get a thank you?

Who is this mystery person, you wonder? They're someone a bit like you. They've got dreams, they're trying to stay healthy and active, and they could use a pointer or two, just like we all could at times.

I have this big goal: to make staying fit and healthy something everyone can do, regardless of age. But to spread that message far and wide, I need a little help from friends like you.

Here's the scoop: folks often decide on a book based on what others say about it. That means your thoughts could really help someone else—maybe a grandparent, a neighbor, or even a friend you haven't met yet.

Could you take a minute to share your thoughts on our book?

Your words don't cost a penny and will take less than a minute, but they could help another person in a big way. Your review might be the little nudge that helps...

...another senior stay fit and fabulous.
   ...a grandparent play with their grandkids without any aches.
   ...someone find a new favorite way to stay active.
   ...a future Pilates pro get their start.
   ...and maybe even spark a new passion.

Ready to spread some kindness? Just scan the QR below to leave your review:

   If you're the kind of person who gets a kick out of doing good, guess what? You're our kind of person, too. Welcome to the family!

And hey, as you flip through the following pages, I'm super excited to show you how to weave Pilates into your day-to-day life in ways that are super simple and totally doable. You're going to love the tips and tricks waiting for you!

A huge thank you from me. Now, let's get back to the fun stuff!

- Your biggest cheerleader, Eva Strong

P.S. - Here's a little secret: when you share something awesome with someone else, it doesn't just help them—it makes you shine, too. If you think this book could make another person's day brighter, why not pass it along?

4

DIVERSIFYING YOUR PILATES TOOLKIT

Imagine opening a well-loved cookbook to find pages filled with new, unexplored dishes from around the world beyond the familiar recipes you've tried and loved. Each recipe offers different flavors, techniques, and outcomes, expanding your culinary skills and palate. This chapter serves a similar purpose for your Pilates practice. Here, we'll explore the Pilates "equipment kitchen," filled with tools that add depth, challenge, and variety to your routine, much like new recipes would to your cooking repertoire.

Introduction to Pilates Apparatus

Pilates isn't just mat exercises; it's a whole world of specialized equipment designed to enhance and diversify your practice. With its sliding carriage and resistance springs, the Reformer brings a dynamic challenge to workouts, allowing for a wide range of motion and the ability to work against resistance in new ways. The Cadillac, also known as the Trapeze Table, is like a Pilates playground, offering support for advanced stretches and strengthening exercises with its bars, springs, and straps. Then there's the Wunda Chair, a compact but versatile piece of equipment that intensifies core exercises and balance work. Each apparatus opens up new possibilities, helping to target specific muscle groups, improve balance, and increase flexibility with precision and support.

Adapting Equipment for Seniors

While Pilates equipment offers numerous benefits, it's crucial to adapt these tools for senior practitioners, focusing on safety and the most beneficial outcomes. For instance, the Reformer can be set at a higher elevation to make getting on and off easier for those with mobility issues. Exercises can also be modified to be gentler, focusing on range of motion rather than resistance. Similarly, the Cadillac can be used for supported stretches that might be challenging on the mat, reducing the risk of overstretching or injury. The key is to start slowly, familiarizing oneself with each piece of equipment under the guidance of a certified Pilates instructor who can tailor exercises to individual needs and limitations.

Home Alternatives to Pilates Equipment

Only some have access to a fully-equipped Pilates studio, but you can still enjoy the benefits of apparatus-based exercises. Many household items can serve as effective substitutes. For example, a sturdy chair can mimic the support and functionality of the Wunda Chair for seated exercises. Resistance bands or a pair of tights can replace Reformer springs for resistance work. Even a broomstick held between your hands can simulate the bar work done on the Cadillac, helping with upper body stretches and balance exercises. These DIY solutions make advanced Pilates practice accessible and affordable, allowing you to enjoy various exercises from the comfort of your home.

When to Integrate Equipment into Practice

Adding equipment to your Pilates practice isn't about making exercises harder; it's about making them more effective and tailored to your body's needs. But when is the right time to introduce these tools? The answer hinges on a solid foundation of Pilates principles and techniques learned on the mat. Once you're comfortable with basic exercises and understand how to engage your core, maintain proper alignment, and move with control and precision, you might be ready to explore the added challenge and support that equipment can offer. It's also wise to consult a Pilates instructor who can assess your readiness and safely integrate equipment into your routine.

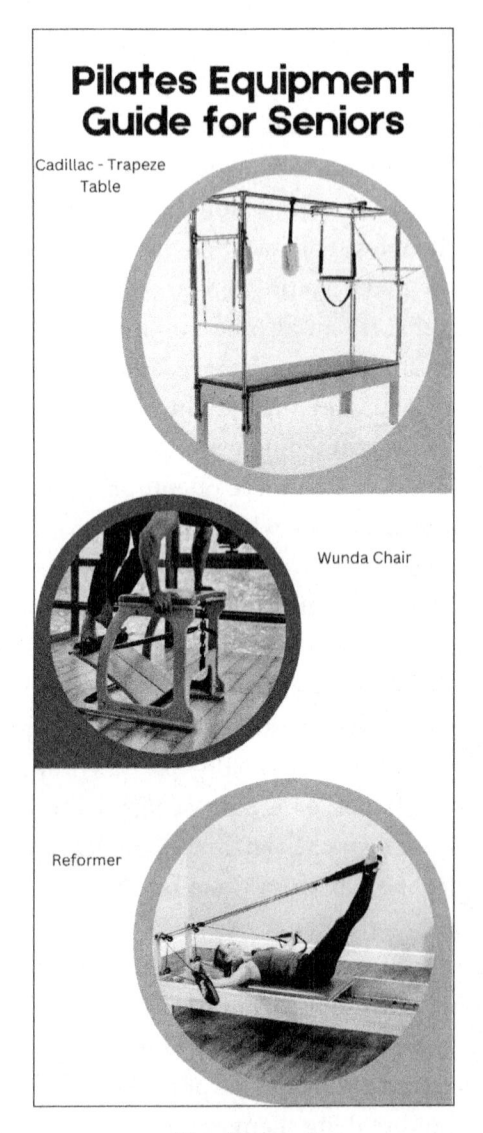

Pilates Equipment

AM I READY FOR PILATES EQUIPMENT?

A Checklist for Seniors

Moving to Pilates equipment exercises represents an exciting step in your fitness journey, offering new challenges and benefits. This checklist is designed to help seniors evaluate their readiness to safely and effectively incorporate Pilates equipment into their routines.

Physical Readiness

[ ] **Consistent Practice:** Have I been consistently practicing Pilates mat exercises for at least 3-6 months?

[ ] **Core Strength:** Do I feel my core strength has improved significantly since I started Pilates?

[ ] **Flexibility:** Have I noticed improvements in my flexibility and range of motion?

[ ] **Balance:** Am I more stable performing standing or balancing exercises than when I began?

[ ] **Injury-Free:** Am I currently free from injuries that could be exacerbated by using Pilates equipment?

Health Considerations

[ ] **Doctor's Approval:** Has my doctor or healthcare provider given me the green light to increase my physical activity level?

[ ] **Chronic Conditions:** If I have chronic conditions (like arthritis, osteoporosis, or heart disease), have I discussed moving to equipment-based exercises with a healthcare professional?

[ ] **Pain Management:** Do I understand how to differentiate between good pain (muscle fatigue) and bad pain (injury or strain)?

Knowledge and Support

[ ] **Understanding of Equipment:** Do I have a basic understanding of Pilates equipment and its purpose?

[ ] **Access to Instruction:** Do I have access to a certified Pilates instructor who can introduce me to equipment safely?

[ ] **Safety Measures:** Am I familiar with safety measures and proper form when using Pilates equipment?

. . .

Personal Commitment

[ ] **Time and Frequency:** Am I willing and able to dedicate more time to my Pilates practice, including sessions with equipment?

[ ] **Learning Attitude:** Am I open to learning new Pilates exercises and possibly facing challenges as I adjust to the equipment?

[ ] **Financial Investment:** Am I prepared for the potential financial investment in classes, sessions, or personal equipment?

Goals and Motivation

[ ] **Clear Objectives:** Do I have clear fitness goals that I believe Pilates equipment exercises will help me achieve?

[ ] **Self-Motivation:** Am I motivated to challenge myself and take my Pilates practice to the next level?

[ ] **Long-Term Vision:** Do I see Pilates equipment exercises as a long-term addition to my fitness routine?

If you've checked most of the boxes, you might be ready to explore the exciting world of Pilates equipment! Starting slow and working with a certified instructor can ensure a safe and enjoyable transition.

Pilates Equipment Manufactures and DIY Alternatives

Pilates Equipment Manufacturers

1. Balanced Body - Renowned for their quality and innovation, Balanced Body offers a wide range of Pilates equipment, including reformers, chairs, and studio accessories.

2. STOTT PILATES by Merrithew - Provides premium Pilates equipment focused on ergonomics and precise movement. Their product line spans from reformers to smaller accessories like stability balls.

3. Pilates Designs - Known for handcrafted, durable equipment, Pilates Designs produces reformers and other apparatuses suitable for both studio and home use.

4. Peak Pilates - Offering a blend of classic craftsmanship and modern innovation, Peak Pilates has a comprehensive selection of equipment, including eco-friendly reformers.

5. Gratz - Celebrated for their adherence to the original designs and specifications of Joseph Pilates himself, making their equipment a favorite among classical Pilates enthusiasts.

DIY Alternatives for Home Practice

1. For the Reformer: Sliding Furniture Pads - Use sliding furniture pads or gliders on a carpeted surface to mimic the sliding motion of a reformer carriage for exercises like leg slides and planks.

2. For the Pilates Chair: Sturdy Chair and Resistance Bands - A sturdy dining chair can substitute for a Pilates chair. Combine with resistance bands attached to the chair legs for added resistance in exercises like seated leg presses.

3. For the Cadillac: Resistance Bands and Pull-Up Bar - Install a pull-up bar in a doorway and attach resistance bands to simulate a Cadillac's trapeze and spring functionalities for arm and leg exercises.

4. For the Magic Circle: Resistance Band Loop - A looped resistance band can replicate the tension exercises of the Magic Circle, offering flexibility and resistance training for the inner and outer thighs, arms, and chest.

5. For the Barrel: Large Stability Ball - A large stability ball can serve as an alternative to the Pilates barrel, supporting the spine and assisting in stretching exercises to increase back flexibility and strength.

Additional Resources

Pilates Method Alliance (PMA) - The PMA website is a great resource for finding certified instructors and studios, which often have recommendations for equipment suppliers or local DIY tips.

Online Marketplaces - Websites like Amazon, eBay, and Craigslist can be sources for both new and used Pilates equipment, offering options for various budgets.

Pilates Instructional Videos and Books - Look for resources that offer equipment setup guides, maintenance tips, and usage instructions to maximize the benefits of your Pilates practice, whether you're using manufactured equipment or DIY alternatives.

When choosing equipment, consider your space, budget, and specific Pilates practice needs. Always prioritize safety, especially when opting for DIY solutions, to ensure a productive, injury-free practice.

Exploring the diverse world of Pilates equipment, we unlock new dimensions of our practice, like discovering new recipes that can transform our cooking. Each apparatus offers unique benefits, challenging and supporting our bodies in ways mat exercises alone cannot. By adapting these tools for senior use and finding creative home alternatives, we ensure that everyone can enjoy the richness of a diversified Pilates practice, regardless of age or access to a studio.

4.1 CHAIR PILATES: AN ACCESSIBLE ALTERNATIVE FOR ENHANCED MOBILITY

Chair Pilates emerges as a beacon of inclusivity in the Pilates landscape, extending the practice's benefits to those who may find traditional mat exercises challenging. This adaptation of Pilates not only ensures accessibility but also maintains the core principles of control, precision, and flow, making it an ideal choice for seniors aiming to enhance their mobility, strength, and balance.

Benefits of Chair Pilates

Chair Pilates offers a gentle yet effective way to engage the body, particularly beneficial for individuals with limited mobility or balance concerns. Here's why it stands out:

- **Safety and Stability**: The chair provides a stable base, reducing the risk of falls during exercise, a crucial consideration for seniors.
- **Adaptability**: Exercises can be easily modified to suit varying fitness levels, ensuring everyone can participate and benefit.
- **Improved Posture**: By focusing on core strength and spinal alignment, chair Pilates helps improve posture, alleviating common aches and pains.
- **Enhanced Mobility**: Regular practice increases flexibility and range of motion, contributing to easier movement in daily tasks.

Core Chair Exercises

Various exercises can be performed using a chair, targeting the whole body. Here are a few to get started:

- **Seated Leg Lifts**: Sit tall with feet flat on the floor. Slowly lift one leg at a time, keeping the core engaged. This strengthens the legs and abdominal muscles.

GENTLE WALL PILATES FOR SENIORS:

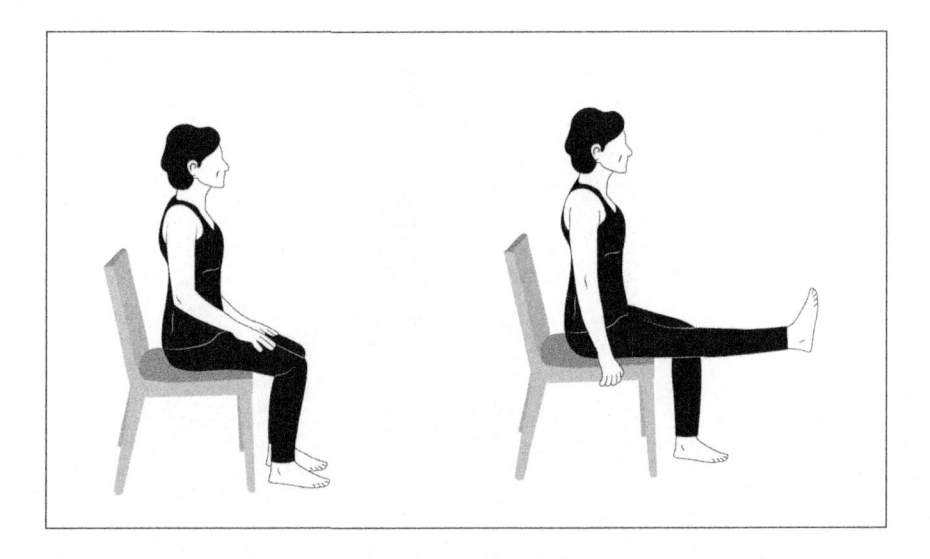

- **Arm Circles:** Extend your arms to the sides at shoulder height. Circle them slowly to improve shoulder mobility and strengthen arm muscles.

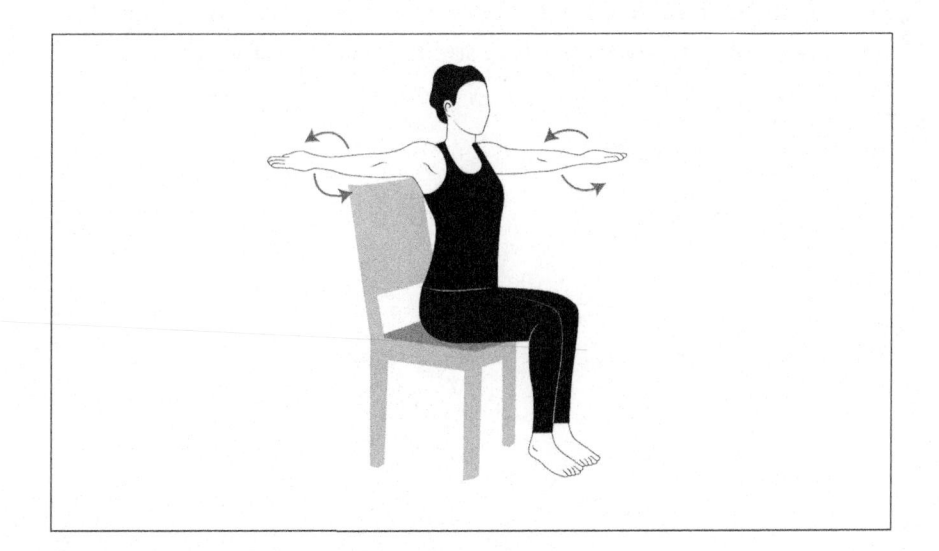

- **Spine Twist:** Sit at the edge of the chair, feet planted firmly. Twist your torso to one side, holding the back of the chair for support, then switch. This movement enhances spinal flexibility.

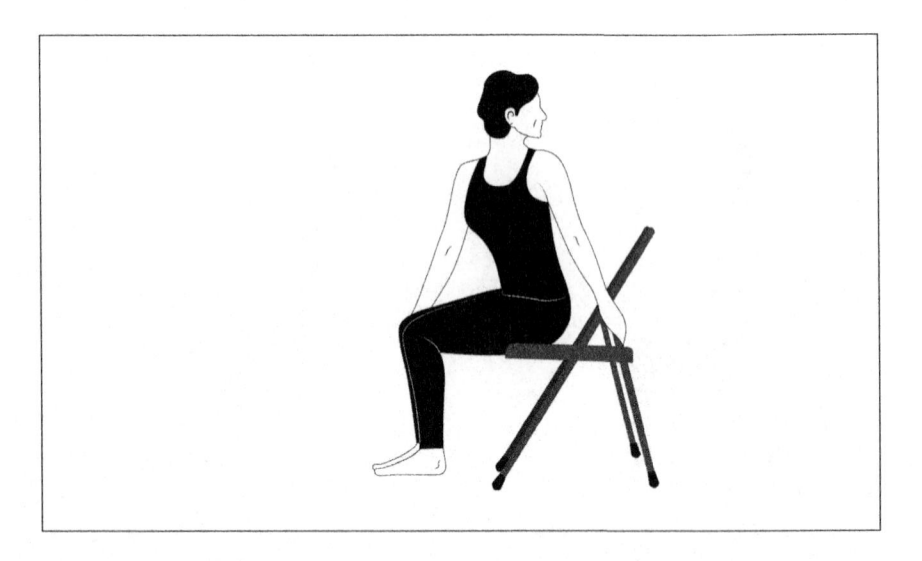

Incorporating Props

To add variety and intensity to your chair Pilates routine, consider integrating simple props:

• **Resistance Bands:** Place a band under your feet while seated for leg presses, offering resistance that strengthens leg muscles.

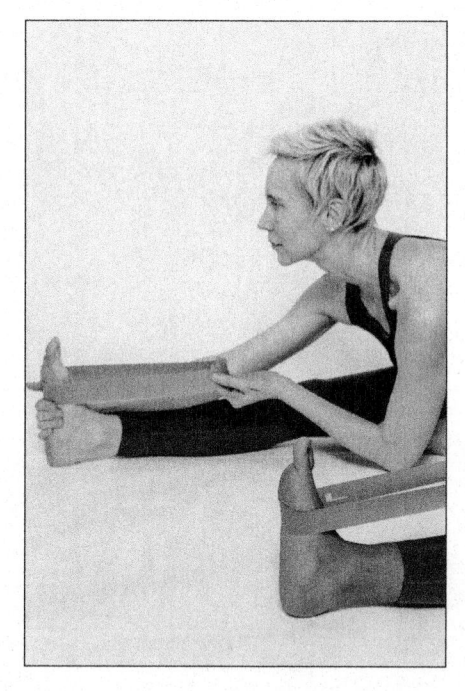

Resistance Bands

• **Pilates Balls:** Holding a small ball with both hands while doing arm lifts or twists engages and strengthens the core and upper body muscles.

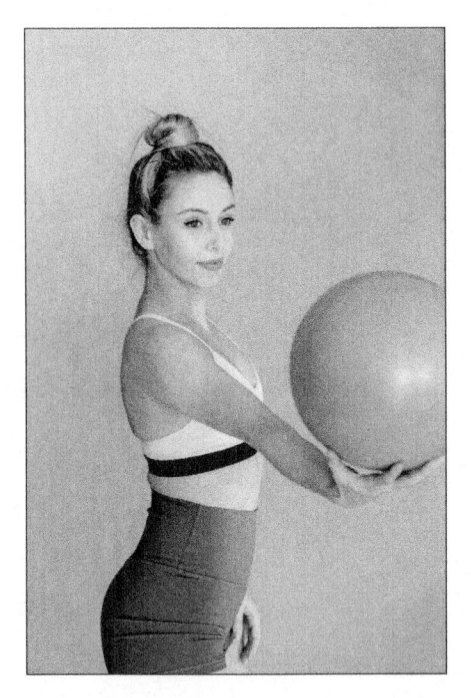

Pilates Ball

• **Foam Rollers:** Place a foam roller vertically along the back of the chair to support and align the spine during exercises, enhancing posture and balance.

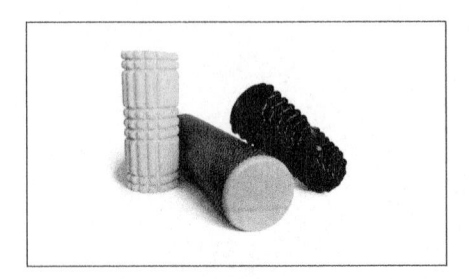

Foam Rollers

Creating a Comprehensive Chair Routine

Crafting a balanced routine involves selecting exercises that work for all major muscle groups, promoting overall well-being. Here's a structure to follow:

- **Warm-Up:** Begin with gentle neck and shoulder rolls to loosen up the muscles and joints.
- **Strength and Flexibility:** Incorporate exercises like seated leg lifts and spine twists, focusing on controlled movements to build strength and enhance flexibility.
- **Balance and Coordination:** Use props like balls for grip exercises, improving hand-eye coordination and balance.
- **Cool Down:** Finish with deep breathing and gentle stretches to relax the muscles and center the mind.

This chair Pilates routine offers a comprehensive approach, ensuring a well-rounded practice that strengthens, stretches, and balances the body. With regular practice, you'll notice improvements in mobility, strength, and overall vitality, making everyday movements smoother and more enjoyable.

4.2 COMBINING PILATES WITH OTHER LOW-IMPACT EXERCISES

The beauty of Pilates lies in its flexibility and how well it plays with other forms of exercise. This synergy enriches our physical regimen and keeps our minds engaged and our bodies guessing. From the serene stretches of Yoga to the fluid movements of Tai Chi and the buoyant resistance of Aquatic exercises, blending Pilates with these practices creates a holistic workout routine that caters to every aspect of our well-being.

Synergizing Pilates with Yoga

Imagine the strength and control of Pilates meeting the flexibility and mindfulness of Yoga. This combination is like a dance, where each discipline complements the other, creating a routine that balances strength with flexibility. Here's how you can weave Yoga into your Pilates sessions:

- **Start with a Yoga warm-up:** Use Yoga poses like Cat-Cow or Mountain pose to warm up your body. This prepares your muscles and joints and centers your mind for the Pilates workout ahead.

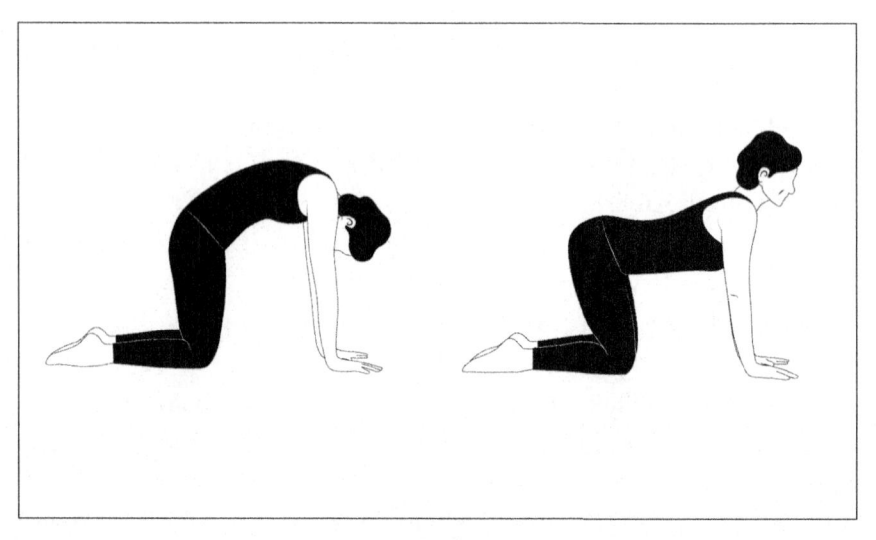

Cat-Cow

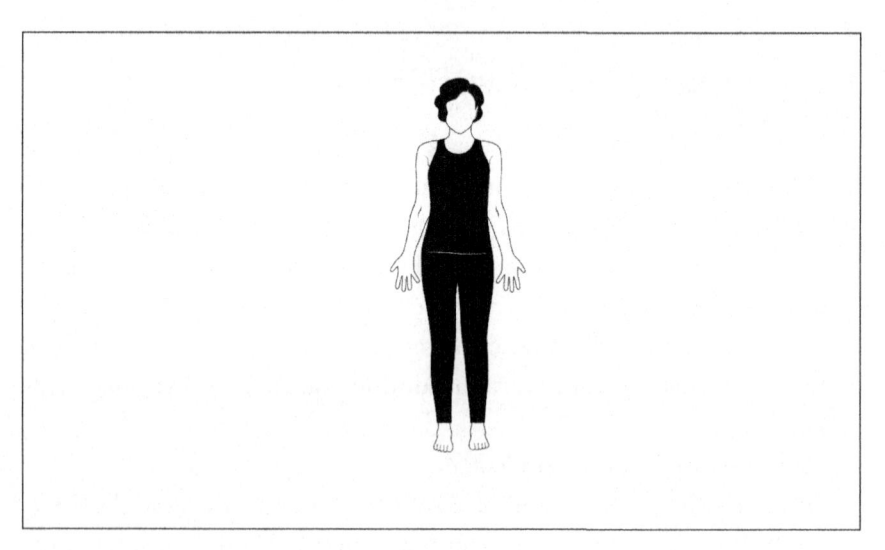

Mountain Pose

- **Incorporate Yoga poses for flexibility**: After a series of Pilates exercises, integrate Yoga poses such as the Downward Dog or Pigeon pose. These poses enhance the flexibility work of Pilates, stretching out muscles that have been activated during your session.

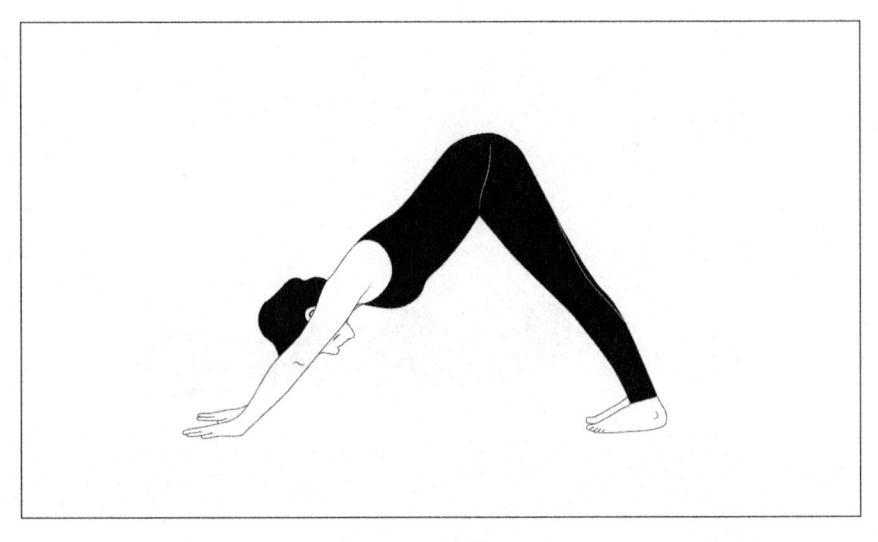

Downward Dog

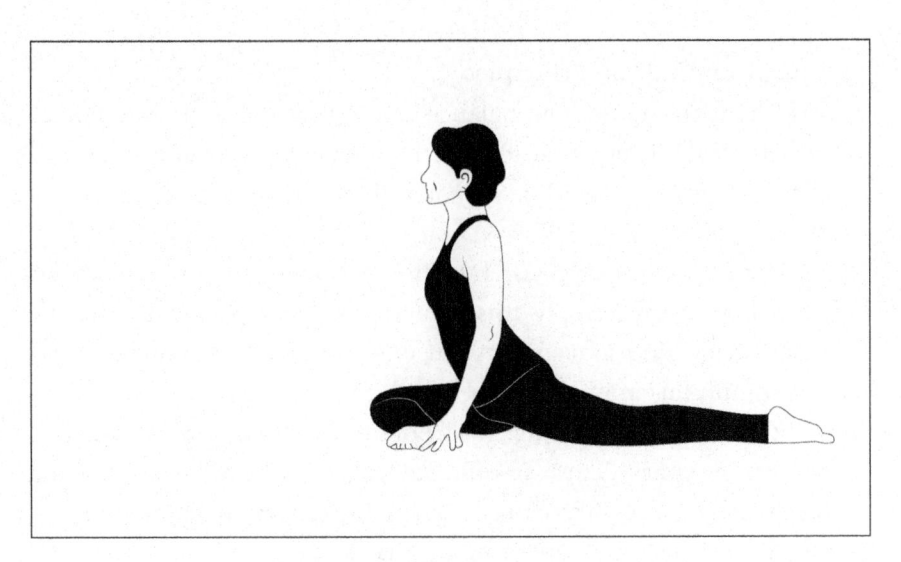

Pigeon Pose

- **End with Yoga relaxation:** Conclude your routine with Yoga's Savasana or a seated meditation to relax the body deeply and assimilate the benefits of your workout.

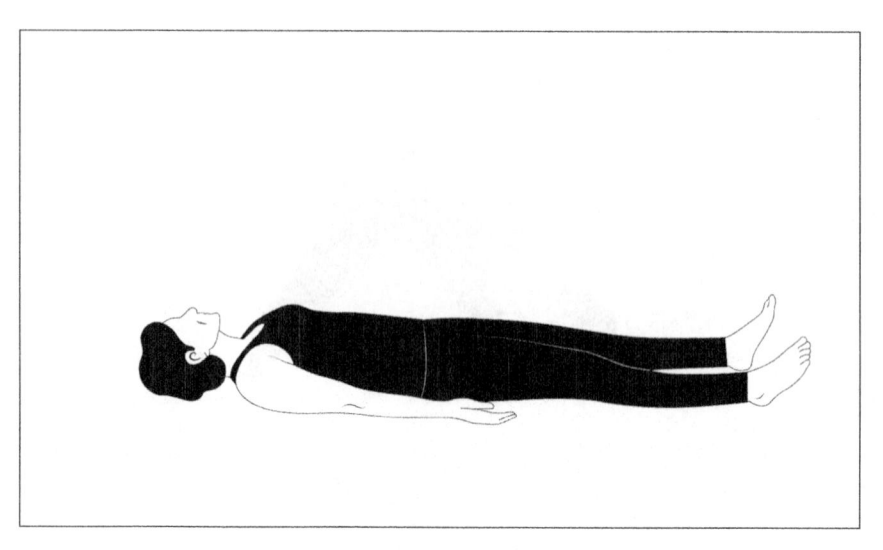

Savasana

Integrating Tai Chi Principles

Tai Chi, focusing on flow, balance, and mindfulness, adds a dimension of graceful movement to Pilates that enhances proprioception and equilibrium. Here's how Tai Chi principles can enrich your Pilates practice:

• **Flow between exercises:** Tai Chi emphasizes smooth transitions between movements. Apply this principle to your Pilates routine by focusing on flowing gracefully from one exercise to the next, maintaining continuous movement and breath control.

• **Balance and grounding:** Incorporate Tai Chi's balance exercises before or after your Pilates workout. Standing on one leg or performing Tai Chi's 'wave hands like clouds' can improve your balance, stability, and focus, which is essential for many Pilates exercises.

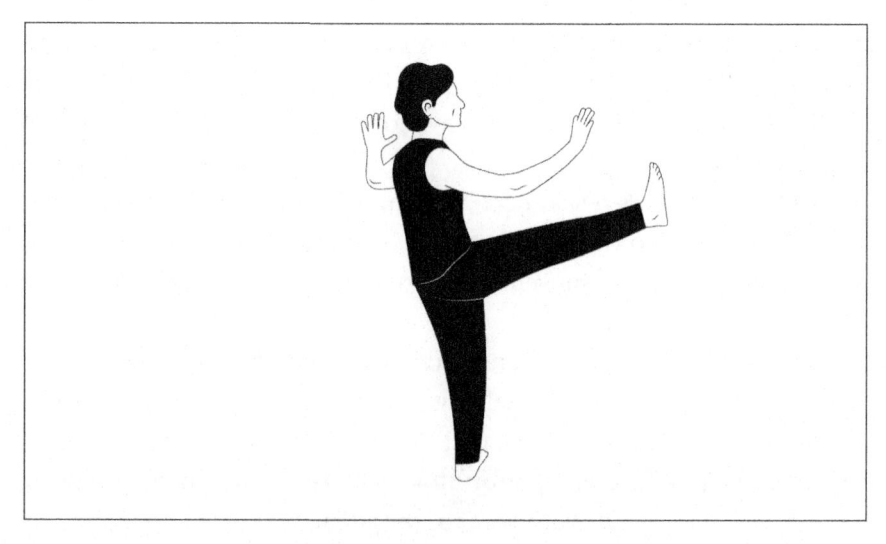

Standing on One Leg

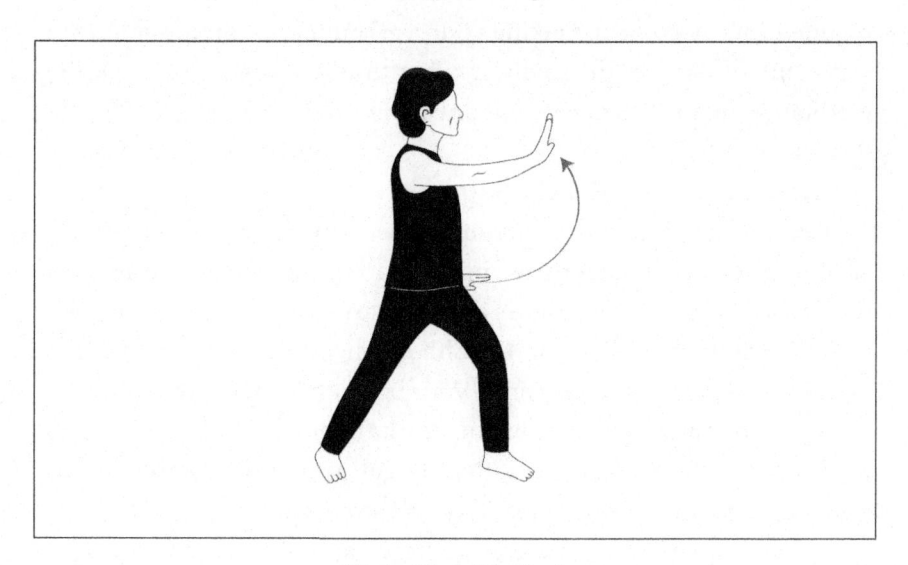

Waving Hands Like Clouds

- **Mindfulness and breath:** Let the mindful breathing and present-moment awareness of Tai Chi infuse your Pilates practice. Focus on breathing deeply and being fully present in each movement, enhancing the mind-body connection.

Aquatic Pilates

Aquatic Pilates, or Poolates, is Pilates performed in the water, offering the benefits of buoyancy and resistance. The water supports your body, making exercises easier on the joints, while the resistance challenges your muscles in new ways. Here's how to take advantage of Aquatic Pilates:

- **Use the water's resistance:** Perform Pilates exercises like leg kicks, arm circles, or torso twists in the water. The water's resistance increases the intensity of these movements, strengthening your muscles more effectively.
- **Buoyancy for support and challenge:** The water's buoyancy can support your body during challenging exercises, making them accessible if you have balance concerns. Conversely, you can use this buoyancy as a challenge by performing exercises like floating planks, requiring you to engage your core to stay afloat.
- **Cooling and soothing:** The water's cool temperature can help regulate your body heat, making your workout more comfortable, especially on hot days. Additionally, moving through water has a soothing, meditative quality that can enhance the stress-reducing benefits of Pilates.

Crafting a Mixed-Modal Routine

Creating a routine incorporating Pilates with other low-impact exercises ensures a comprehensive approach to fitness, keeping your workouts varied and engaging. Here's a simple structure to get you started:

- **Warm up with Yoga or Tai Chi:** Begin with gentle Yoga stretches or Tai Chi movements to warm up your body and center your mind.
- **Core Pilates work:** Move on to the main part of your routine, focusing on Pilates exercises that target your core, improve your posture, and enhance your flexibility and strength.
- **Add Aquatic Exercises:** If you have access to a pool, include a session of Aquatic Pilates once a week to benefit from the resistance and buoyancy of water.
- **Cool down and stretch:** Conclude your routine with Yoga poses focused on flexibility and relaxation, allowing your body to recover and absorb the benefits of your workout.

By blending Pilates with Yoga, Tai Chi, and Aquatic exercises, you create a rich, diversified fitness regimen that addresses all physical and mental health aspects. This holistic approach keeps your body challenged, your mind engaged, and your spirit uplifted, ensuring that your journey to wellness is as rewarding as it is effective.

4.3 ADVANCED STRETCHING TECHNIQUES FOR FLEXIBILITY

In the realm of Pilates, flexibility is not just about reaching your toes; it's about creating a symphony of movement that allows your body to perform at its peak. When woven into your Pilates fabric, advanced stretching techniques can elevate this performance, granting you a range of motion that easily dances between strength and suppleness. This segment explores the sophisticated world of stretching, guiding you through dynamic and static stretches, the transformative power of Proprioceptive Neuromuscular Facilitation (PNF), and the critical journey of stretching safely.

Beyond Basic Stretching

Introducing advanced stretching techniques into your Pilates regimen opens doors to new levels of flexibility and motion. These aren't mere stretches; they're strategic movements designed with a deeper understanding of the body's mechanics. Here, we venture into stretches that lengthen and fortify the muscles, ensuring every fiber moves harmoniously.

Dynamic vs. Static Stretching

The debate between dynamic and static stretching finds its resolution in the balanced approach of Pilates. Dynamic stretches involve movement and momentum to stretch the muscles and prepare the body for the activity ahead. In contrast, static stretches hold a position for a period, cool the body down, and deepen the flexibility attained.

- **Dynamic Stretching**: Perfect for the start of your Pilates session, these stretches might include leg swings or arm circles. They gently wake the muscles, signaling them to prepare for the work ahead, enhancing blood flow and reducing the risk of injury.
- **Static Stretching**: These come into play after the core of your Pilates practice. Imagine holding a leg stretch or a torso twist, feeling the muscle gently extend under your sustained attention. This method

helps in cooling down and deepens the stretches achieved during your session.

PNF Stretching for Pilates

PNF stretching stands as a bridge between passive stretching and active muscle engagement. This technique, which utilizes the contraction and stretching of muscles, is a game-changer in improving flexibility and strength. Here's how it blends beautifully with Pilates:

- **Contract-Relax:** After moving into a stretch, you gently contract the muscle for a few seconds, then relax deeper into the stretch. This method can be applied to leg stretches on the Pilates reformer, where a gentle contraction is followed by a deeper release after reaching a point of tension.
- **Hold-Relax with Agonist Contraction:** This variation involves a stretch, a muscle contraction, and then stretching further while activating the opposing muscle group. It's particularly effective in Pilates for deepening stretches like the hamstring stretch, promoting flexibility and muscular balance.

Safety and Progression in Stretching

As we tread the path of advanced stretching, the signposts of safety and progression ensure a journey that enhances our practice without veering into the realm of injury. Here's what to keep in mind:

- **Warm-Up Is Non-Negotiable:** A thorough warm-up is crucial before delving into advanced stretches. Engage in light, dynamic stretches or a few minutes of gentle Pilates movements to prepare the body.
- **Listen to Your Body:** The language of discomfort is your guide. While stretching should challenge you, it should never cause pain. If a stretch feels too intense, ease back and approach it gradually.
- **Incremental Progression:** Gradual progression is the key to safely incorporating advanced stretches. Increase the intensity or duration of stretches bit by bit, allowing your body to adapt without strain.
- **Consultation and Guidance:** When experimenting with techniques like PNF, consulting with a Pilates instructor or a physical therapist ensures you apply the methods correctly, tailored to your body's needs and capabilities.

Incorporating advanced stretching techniques into your Pilates practice is like tuning a musical instrument. Each stretch, carefully chosen and executed, enhances your body's harmony, allowing for a performance that resonates with strength, flexibility, and grace. Through dynamic and static stretching, the targeted approach of PNF, and a commitment to safe progression, your Pilates journey unfolds into an evermore fluid and expansive dance of movement.

4.4 THE ROLE OF RESISTANCE BANDS IN PILATES PROGRESSION

Imagine discovering a versatile and adaptable tool that enhances your Pilates workouts and propels your fitness journey forward with vibrant new challenges. Resistance bands are precisely that magical ingredient in the world of Pilates, offering a spectrum of benefits and applications that can significantly enrich your practice. These stretchy strips of rubber, ranging from thin, light bands to thicker, more robust versions, introduce a level of resistance that can be adjusted to suit your strength and flexibility, making them an ideal companion for Pilates enthusiasts at any stage.

Introduction to Resistance Bands

Resistance bands come in various types, each offering unique benefits. The most common include loop bands, which form a continuous circle and are perfect for lower body exercises; therapy bands, which are thinner and designed for rehabilitation; and tube bands with handles, offering a grip for upper body exercises. Their primary appeal lies in their ability to add resistance without needing heavy weights, engaging muscles more deeply and effectively. This resistance not only aids in building strength but also improves flexibility and joint mobility, making bands a multifaceted tool in the Pilates arsenal.

Incorporating Bands into Pilates Routines

Incorporating resistance bands into your Pilates routine adds a layer of challenge and excitement. Here are a few ways to weave them into your practice:

• **Leg Presses:** While lying on your back, loop a band around your foot and press against the resistance as you extend and bend your leg. This exercise targets the quadriceps and hamstrings.

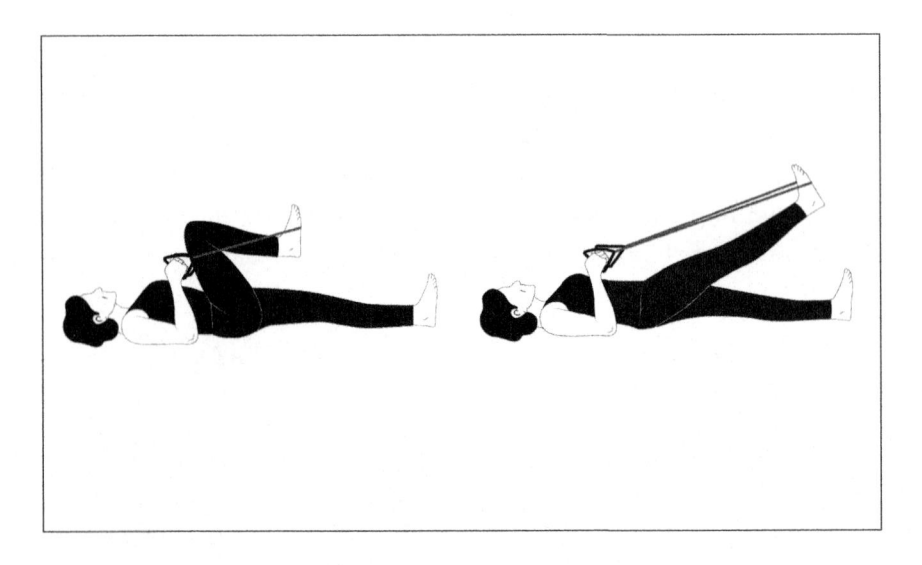

- **Arm Toning:** Holding the ends of a band, perform arm curls or shoulder presses. The band's resistance helps tone and strengthen the arms and shoulders.

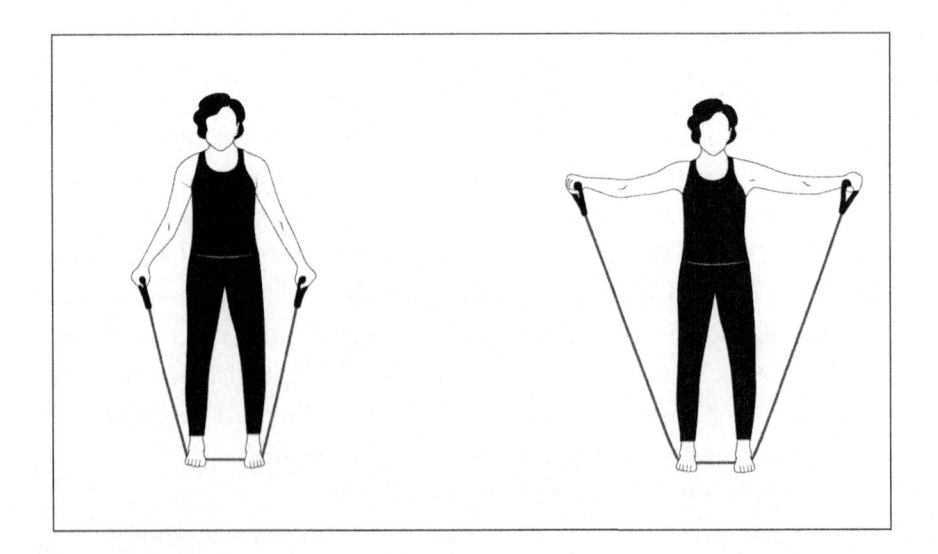

- **Core Strengthening:** Wrap a band around your back or a solid pole while doing sit-ups or twists. The added resistance challenges your core muscles, enhancing strength and stability.

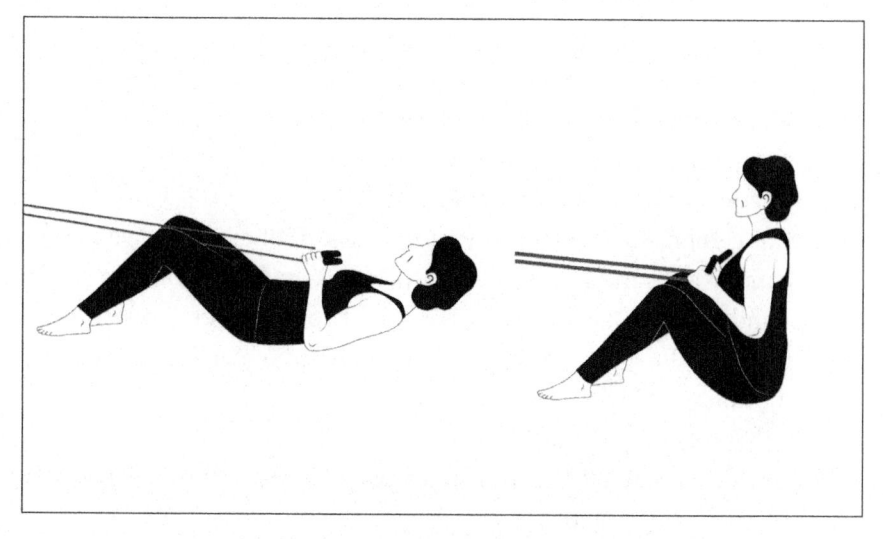

Sit-Ups with Resistance Band

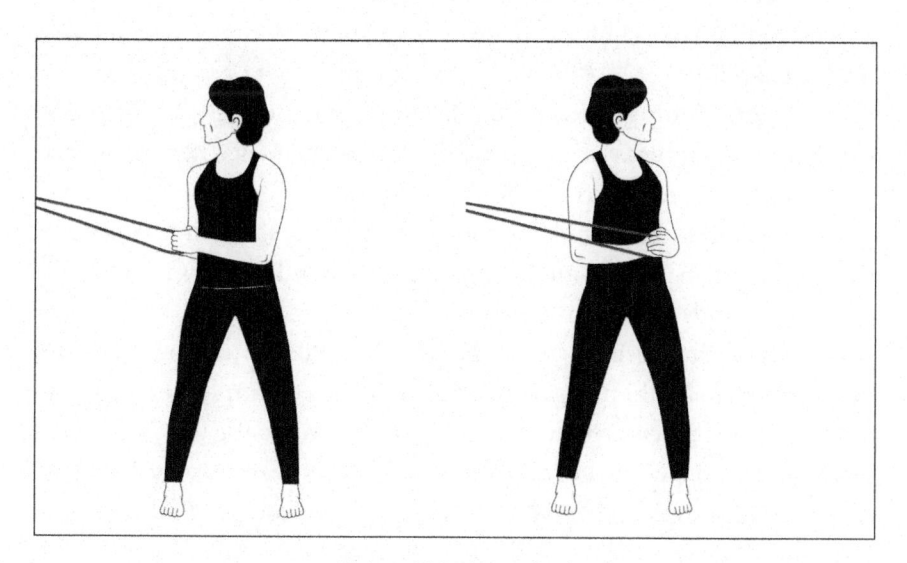

Twists with Resistance Band

These examples barely scratch the surface. With creativity, almost any Pilates exercise can be adapted to include a resistance band, adding depth and variety to your workouts.

Customizing Resistance for Individual Needs

The key to effectively using resistance bands lies in selecting the right resistance level. Start with a lighter band, gradually moving to thicker bands as your strength improves. Pay attention to your body's feedback. If an exercise feels too easy, it might be time to progress to a band with more resistance. Conversely, switch to a lighter band if you struggle to maintain proper form. This tailored approach ensures a safe, effective workout that grows with you.

Advancements should be measured and deliberate. As you grow more comfortable and stronger, intersperse exercises with higher resistance bands, but always prioritize form and control over the resistance level. This careful progression fosters a deepening of Pilates practice that is both rewarding and sustainable.

Band Safety and Maintenance

To ensure a safe and enjoyable experience with resistance bands, consider these best practices:

- **Regular Inspection:** Before each use, check your bands for signs of wear or damage, such as small tears or thinning areas, which could lead to snapping.
- **Proper Storage:** Keep bands away from direct sunlight and extreme temperatures to prevent degradation. Storing them in a cool, dry place helps prolong their life.
- **Correct Usage:** Avoid snapping or releasing the bands forcefully. Control is key in Pilates, and this principle extends to how you handle resistance bands to prevent injury.

Incorporating resistance bands into your Pilates routine opens up possibilities for enhancing your practice. These simple yet powerful tools introduce new challenges and variety, allowing for a tailored workout experience that can evolve with your fitness journey. Whether you're looking to deepen your strength, improve your flexibility, or add a refreshing twist to your routines, resistance bands offer a pathway to achieving these goals gracefully and effectively.

4.5 PILATES SEQUENCES FOR EVERY SEASON OF THE YEAR

The year's rhythm brings with it a symphony of changes, from the budding promises of spring to the serene quiet of winter. Each season invites us to adapt and tune our Pilates practice to its unique tempo, transforming our routine into a reflection of the world around us. This adaptation keeps our practice fresh and engaging and aligns our physical activity with the natural cycles, enhancing our connection to our bodies and the environment.

Seasonal Adaptations in Practice

Adapting your Pilates practice to the changing seasons involves more than just switching up routines. It's about responding to the body's natural inclinations during different times of the year, taking advantage of each season's energy and mood. For instance, the revitalizing air of spring might inspire more dynamic awakening exercises, while the reflective ambiance of winter calls for routines that warm and invigorate from within.

Spring Renewal Routines

As nature reawakens, so does our need for a movement that rejuvenates and energizes. Spring routines focus on awakening muscles that have been in hibernation, gently encouraging flexibility and strength.

- Start with gentle stretches that mimic the unfolding of leaves and flowers, such as spine stretches and arm reaches, to loosen the body.
- Incorporate exercises that build foundational strength for more active summer months ahead, like planks and leg circles, to awaken the core and lower body.
- Use breathwork to invigorate the body further, drawing in the fresh energy of spring with each inhale.

Summer Strength and Stamina

The warmth and vitality of summer offer the perfect backdrop for building strength and endurance. With longer days and abundant energy, focus on routines that challenge and fortify.

- Intensify your practice with resistance bands or weights to add a strengthening component to traditional Pilates moves.
- Incorporate longer sequences that require stamina, such as repeated sun salutations adapted to Pilates, to take advantage of high energy levels.
- Practice outdoors whenever possible, allowing the sun's warmth to deepen stretches and enhance the mood-lifting benefits of your routine.

Fall Flexibility Focus

As the days begin to shorten and the air cools, focus on maintaining flexibility and grounding your energy in preparation for the winter.

• Emphasize stretches that target the whole body, focusing on fluid movements that mimic the falling leaves, such as roll-downs and windmill arms.

• Introduce balance exercises like single-leg stands or the Pilates saw, mirroring the balancing act between the seasons.

• Adapt your breathwork to slow, deep breathing, reflecting the calming nature of autumn and preparing the body and mind for the introspection of winter.

Winter Warm-Up Workouts

The chill of winter calls for routines that warm the body from the inside out, boosting circulation and combating the sedentary tendencies of colder weather.

• Begin each session with a warm-up that includes dynamic movements to generate heat, such as marching in place or gentle jogging on the spot.

• Focus on core-strengthening exercises that build internal heat and support the spine, like bridges and tabletop leg presses.

• Integrate props such as foam rollers for self-massage, encouraging blood flow and providing soothing warmth to stiff muscles.

By thoughtfully adapting our Pilates practice to the ebb and flow of the seasons, we keep our routine engaging and responsive to our needs and deepen our connection to the natural world. This harmonious approach ensures our practice remains a dynamic and nurturing part of our lives throughout the year, offering a physical reflection of the world's cycles and rhythms.

4.6 OVERCOMING PLATEAUS: TIPS FOR CONTINUED IMPROVEMENT

Hitting a plateau in your Pilates practice can feel like sailing into a windless sea. You're putting in the effort, but your progress seems to have dropped anchor. It's a common phase for many, indicating that your body has adapted to the current level of challenge. Recognizing and pushing past these still waters requires strategy, patience, and a bit of creativity.

Recognizing a Plateau

Identifying a standstill in your Pilates journey involves tuning into both your physical progress and mental engagement. Signs include:

• Despite regular practice, a noticeable lack of improvement in strength, flexibility, or balance.

• Exercises that once felt challenging now seem routine, with little to no muscle fatigue post-workout.

• A growing sense of monotony or boredom with your sessions, possibly leading to skipped workouts.

Strategies for Breaking Through

Elevating your practice beyond a plateau can rejuvenate your body and enthusiasm for Pilates. Consider these tactics:

• **Introduce New Exercises:** Injecting fresh movements into your routine can awaken different muscle groups and rekindle your interest. Explore variations of familiar exercises or incorporate tools like resistance bands for a new challenge.

• **Adjust Intensity:** Modifying the intensity of your workouts can provide the stimulus your body needs for growth. This could mean increasing the number of repetitions, adding more resistance, or holding poses for longer durations.

• **Seek Advanced Instruction:** A session with a Pilates instructor can provide personalized insights into advancing your practice. They might identify areas for improvement or introduce advanced techniques tailored to your needs.

The Importance of Goal Reassessment

As you navigate the calm of a plateau, it's an opportune time to look at your map and reassess your destination. Goals set at the beginning of your Pilates voyage might no longer align with your current position or aspirations. Reevaluating your goals ensures they remain relevant and challenging. Steps include:

• Reflect on your achievements and how your interests or needs might have evolved.

• Set new targets that stretch your capabilities but are still within reach. This could involve mastering a complex sequence or improving your flexibility to a specific degree.

• Break down these goals into actionable, short-term objectives to maintain a clear direction and sense of progress.

Seeking Inspiration and Support

The voyage through a plateau is one you needn't sail alone. Finding sources of inspiration and support can breathe new life into your practice:

• **Workshops and Retreats**: Attending a Pilates workshop or retreat can expose you to new styles, techniques, and ideas. These experiences can spark inspiration and deepen your practice in unexpected ways.

• **Pilates Communities**: Joining a Pilates community, whether online or in-person, connects you with fellow enthusiasts. Sharing experiences, challenges, and successes can provide motivation and a sense of camaraderie.

• **Inspirational Resources**: Books, documentaries, and online content about Pilates, its history, and its benefits can reignite your passion. Learning about others' transformations through Pilates might just be the wind needed to push past your plateau.

Moving beyond a plateau in your Pilates practice is not just about changing what you do on the mat; it's about shifting your mindset, exploring new territories, and recommitting to your journey with renewed goals and enthusiasm. By recognizing the signs of a standstill, implementing strategies for growth, reassessing your goals, and seeking inspiration and support, you'll find yourself catching a favorable wind, ready to sail towards new horizons in your Pilates adventure.

4.7 PILATES FOR BALANCE AND COORDINATION: ADVANCED TECHNIQUES

Navigating through Pilates practice, one discovers its profound impact on balance and coordination. These elements, vital for our daily activities, can be significantly enhanced through targeted Pilates exercises. This section delves into sophisticated techniques designed to challenge and refine your balance and coordination skills, introducing equipment-based exercises and mindfulness strategies that elevate your Pilates experience.

Advanced Balance Challenges

Elevating your balance through Pilates involves engaging in exercises that push the boundaries of your stability. Here are some innovative ways to intensify your balance work:

- **Single-Leg Variations:** Transform classic Pilates poses by performing them on a single leg. For instance, try a single-leg teaser, where one leg extends into the air as you lift into the teaser position, demanding intense core engagement and balance.

- **Blindfolded Pilates:** Performing familiar exercises with closed eyes drastically changes the challenge, forcing you to rely on proprioception and inner balance. Start with simple poses, gradually moving to more complex sequences.

Coordination with Equipment

Pilates equipment, renowned for its versatility, can be instrumental in advancing your coordination. By incorporating apparatus into your routines, you can explore exercises that demand synchronized movements of different limbs, enhancing your control and precision.

- **Reformer Jump Board:** The jump board attachment for the Reformer introduces a dynamic aspect to your practice. Executing controlled jumps while lying on your back demands harmony between leg movements and core stability.

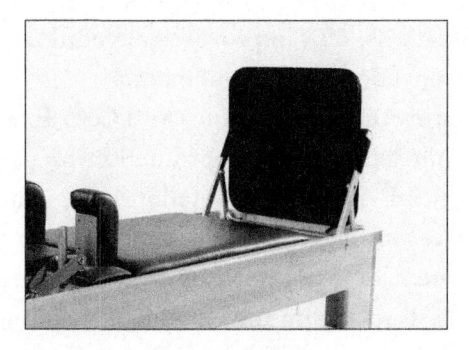

Reformer Jump Board

- **Cadillac Spring Attachments:** Utilize the springs on the Cadillac for arm and leg exercises. Managing the tension while maintaining balance on the table challenges your coordination, engaging multiple muscle groups simultaneously.

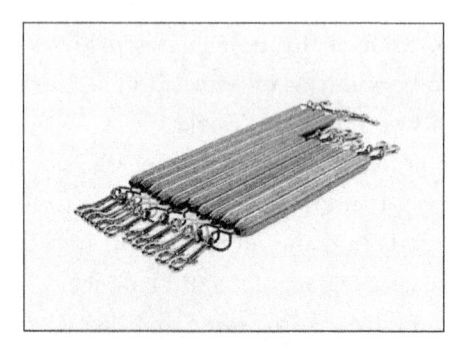

Cadillac Spring Attachments

Incorporating Mindfulness for Improved Coordination

Mindfulness, the practice of maintaining a moment-by-moment awareness of our thoughts, feelings, bodily sensations, and surrounding environment, can be a powerful tool for enhancing coordination in Pilates. Here's how this practice can be integrated:

- **Focused Movement:** Before initiating an exercise, take a moment to visualize the movement in your mind, paying attention to the muscles involved and the sequence of actions. This mental rehearsal primes your body for precise execution.
- **Breath Coordination:** Align your movements with your breath. For instance, synchronize your leg lifts with inhalations and your returns with exhalations. This improves your coordination and deepens the mind-body connection, central to Pilates.

Tracking Improvements in Balance and Coordination

Monitoring your balance and coordination progress can be motivating and insightful, helping you tailor your practice to address specific needs. Here are effective ways to measure your advancements:

- **Balance Time:** Use a stopwatch to time how long you can maintain balance poses. Tracking improvements in how long you can hold a single-leg stand or a teaser on one leg offers tangible evidence of your progress.
- **Coordination Diaries:** Keep a journal detailing your experiences with coordination-intensive exercises. Note the challenges you face and

the improvements over time. Reflecting on these entries can provide insights into how different techniques or modifications affect your coordination.

• **Video Analysis:** Occasionally, film your practice, focusing on exercises that require high levels of balance and coordination. Watching these videos allows you to observe and adjust your form, ensuring your movements are synchronized and fluid.

In weaving advanced balance and coordination techniques into your Pilates repertoire, you stand to gain improved stability and grace in your movements and embark on a deeper exploration of the connection between mind and body. Through the strategic application of Pilates apparatus, the infusion of mindfulness into your practice, and the diligent tracking of your progress, you unlock new dimensions of physical capability, enhancing your Pilates practice and overall quality of life.

4.8 THE FUTURE OF PILATES IN SENIOR FITNESS: TRENDS AND INNOVATIONS

The landscape of Pilates is ever-evolving, much like the ebb and flow of the tides, bringing fresh perspectives and methodologies to the forefront, especially within the realm of senior fitness. This evolution is marked by a blend of tradition and innovation, where Pilates's timeless principles meet the modern world's cutting-edge trends. In this fusion, we find exciting opportunities to enhance and adapt our practice, ensuring that Pilates remains a vital component of senior fitness well into the future.

Emerging Trends in Pilates

In recent years, we've seen a surge in Pilates trends that cater specifically to the needs and preferences of the senior population. Among these, virtual classes have risen in prominence, offering accessibility and convenience previously unimagined. From the comfort of home, seniors can now engage in guided Pilates sessions, connecting with instructors and fellow practitioners across the globe. This digital shift has democratized access to Pilates, breaking down mobility, transportation, and geographic location barriers.

Fusion workouts represent another burgeoning trend, where Pilates is blended with other forms of exercise to create hybrid routines. These combinations vary widely, from Pilates-Yoga (Yogalates) to incorporating dance, aquatic exercises, or resistance training elements. Such fusion workouts are designed not only to break the monotony but also to address a broader range of physical needs, optimizing the benefits of each session.

Innovative equipment has also made its mark, with new tools being developed to enhance the Pilates experience. From modified reformers catering to seniors' specific needs to balance-enhancing devices that make Pilates more accessible, these innovations are expanding the possibilities within Pilates practice, making it more effective, engaging, and safe for older adults.

Technology's Role in Pilates

Technology has become pivotal in reshaping Pilates practice, especially for seniors. In particular, Online platforms and apps have transformed how Pilates is taught, learned, and practiced. These digital tools offer a wealth of resources, from on-demand classes and instructional videos to progress tracking and personalized workout plans. The ability to customize one's practice, receive instant feedback, and track improvements over time has made Pilates more adaptable and personalized.

Moreover, integrating virtual reality (VR) and augmented reality (AR) into Pilates is on the horizon, promising to create immersive workout experiences that can enhance motivation and engagement. By simulating different environments or providing visual cues for alignment and technique, these technologies can revolutionize the way seniors practice Pilates, making it an even more interactive and enriching experience.

Innovations in Senior Fitness

The intersection of Pilates and senior fitness is witnessing remarkable innovations driven by ongoing research and a deeper understanding of aging. One significant development area is exercises and programs designed to enhance mobility and longevity. These tailored routines focus on improving balance, strengthening the muscles around the joints, and increasing flexibility, all of which are crucial for maintaining independence and quality of life in older age.

Additionally, there's growing emphasis on the cognitive benefits of Pilates, with routines being developed to support physical health and stimulate mental acuity. By incorporating elements that challenge the mind, such as complex sequences or coordination tasks, Pilates is used to support cognitive function, memory, and even emotional well-being.

Adapting to Future Changes

Staying adaptable and open to new approaches is key to ensuring that Pilates remains a vibrant and effective practice for seniors. This means being willing to explore new trends, integrate technology into our routines, and embrace innovations that enhance the efficacy of Pilates. It's about balancing the core principles that define Pilates and the evolving techniques and tools that can enhance its impact.

As instructors and practitioners, we must also commit to ongoing education, staying informed about the latest research in senior fitness and Pilates innovations. This continuous learning process allows us to adapt our practice to meet the changing needs of the senior population, ensuring that Pilates continues to be a powerful tool for promoting health, mobility, and vitality.

In navigating the future of Pilates in senior fitness, our guiding star remains the well-being of our practitioners. By blending the wisdom of traditional Pilates with the insights of contemporary trends and innovations, we forge a path forward that honors the past while embracing the future. A spirit of exploration marks this journey as a commitment to adaptability and dedication to enhancing the lives of seniors through the transformative power of Pilates.

4.9 PILATES RETREATS AND WORKSHOPS: DEEPENING YOUR PRACTICE

Attending Pilates retreats and workshops provides an invaluable opportunity to refine your skills, gain new insights, and connect with a broader community of Pilates enthusiasts. These immersive experiences, often led by seasoned instructors, offer a depth of learning beyond regular studio classes, focusing on personalized attention, advanced techniques, and the holistic benefits of Pilates.

The Perks of Going Deeper

- **Personal Growth:** Retreats and workshops offer a chance to focus intensively on your Pilates practice, helping you push past personal boundaries in a supportive environment.
- **Expert Guidance:** Learning from experienced instructors can provide new techniques, corrections, and insights that are hard to come by in larger class settings or online tutorials.
- **Community Connection:** These gatherings are perfect for meeting others who share your passion for Pilates, offering a sense of belonging and mutual encouragement.

Choosing Your Ideal Pilates Adventure

Selecting the right retreat or workshop involves considering several key factors to ensure it aligns with your needs and goals:

- **Instructor Expertise:** Look for events led by instructors with a strong teaching track record, especially those with experience working with seniors or specific health conditions.
- **Program Focus:** Identify retreats and workshops that match your interests, whether mastering specific Pilates apparatus, exploring Pilates for rehabilitation, or focusing on the mind-body connection.
- **Location and Accessibility:** Ensure the venue is accessible, especially if you have mobility concerns. Many retreats are set in tranquil locations that can enhance the learning experience but consider travel ease and accommodation comfort.
- **Class Size:** Smaller groups allow more individualized attention, so check the participant-to-instructor ratio.

Preparing for an Immersive Learning Experience

To make the most out of a Pilates retreat or workshop, a little preparation can go a long way:

- **Physical Prep:** If the event is more intensive than your usual routine, gradually increase your Pilates practice leading up to it to build stamina and flexibility.
- **Goal Setting:** Define what you hope to achieve or learn from the experience. Having clear objectives can help you stay focused and make the most of the opportunity.
- **Pack Smart:** Bring any personal Pilates gear you use, like your mat or resistance bands, and don't forget comfortable clothing that allows for a full range of motion.

Bringing It All Back Home

The true value of a retreat or workshop lies not only in the experience itself but in how you integrate what you've learned into your daily practice:

- **Practice Notes**: During the event, take notes on exercises, corrections, and any insights the instructor shares. These can be invaluable as you continue your Pilates journey at home.
- **Routine Refresh**: Use new exercises and techniques you've learned to refresh your home routine, keeping your practice dynamic and engaging.
- **Community Ties**: Stay in touch with fellow participants and instructors for ongoing support and motivation. Many retreats and workshops have social media groups or email lists.

Incorporating the rich experiences from Pilates retreats and workshops into your regular practice enriches your understanding and keeps the flame of passion for Pilates burning brightly. It's a reminder that Pilates, like life, is a continuous path of learning, growth, and connection. As you weave these new strands of knowledge and camaraderie into the fabric of your Pilates practice, you'll find yourself moving with more confidence, depth, and joy.

As we close this chapter, remember that deepening your Pilates practice through retreats and workshops is not just about advancing your physical capabilities but also about nurturing your mind and spirit, connecting with a like-minded community, and bringing fresh inspiration and energy into your daily life. These experiences serve as stepping stones, guiding you towards a more fulfilling and enriched Pilates journey. As we transition into the next chapter, we carry forward the lessons learned, ready to explore new dimensions of our practice and well-being.

5

EMBRACING A PILATES LIFESTYLE: NOURISHING BODY AND MIND

Imagine Pilates as a beautiful garden you tend to every day. Your movements are the water, breath, and sunlight - both essential for growth. But, just as a garden can't thrive without fertile soil, your Pilates practice is only as strong as the foundation it's built upon. This foundation? Nutrition. The soil enriches your body, ensuring every stretch and pose brings you closer to your wellness goals.

In this chapter, we dig into how your diet is pivotal in supporting your Pilates regimen. Think of it as cultivating a menu that's as balanced and intentional as your practice, tailored to enhance performance, recovery, and overall well-being.

The Role of Nutrition in Pilates

Just as a car needs the right fuel to run smoothly, your body needs the right nutrients to perform at its best during Pilates. Balanced nutrition supports energy levels, muscle repair, and overall health, making it a crucial part of any fitness routine. It's not just about eating healthy; it's about choosing foods that complement your Pilates goals. For instance, lean proteins aid muscle repair after a challenging session, while complex carbohydrates provide the energy to sustain you through your routines.

Nutritional Guidelines for Pilates Practitioners

Navigating the world of nutrition can feel as complex as mastering a new Pilates pose. Here's a simplified guide to keep you nourished and ready to tackle your sessions:

- **Stay Hydrated:** Water is your best friend. It keeps joints lubricated, helps transport nutrients to your cells, and aids in recovery. Aim for at least eight glasses daily, more if you're active.
- **Protein Intake:** Include a source of lean protein in every meal to help repair and build muscle. Think chicken, fish, tofu, legumes, and dairy.
- **Energy Foods:** Opt for whole grains, fruits, and vegetables to keep your energy levels steady. These foods provide the complex carbs your body uses as fuel.
- **Healthy Fats:** Don't avoid fats; just choose the right ones. Avocados, nuts, seeds, and olive oil are great for heart health and can keep you feeling satisfied.

Anti-Inflammatory Foods for Recovery

After a Pilates session, your muscles might feel tender or sore. This is where anti-inflammatory foods come in. They can help reduce inflammation, speed recovery, and prepare you for your next practice. Some top picks include:

- **Berries (Strawberries, Blueberries, Raspberries, Blackberries)**
- **Main Benefit:** Rich in antioxidants and vitamins, berries can reduce inflammation and lower the risk of disease.
- **Fatty Fish (Salmon, Mackerel, Sardines, Anchovies)**
- **Main Benefit:** High in omega-3 fatty acids, fatty fish help reduce inflammation linked to heart disease, cancer, and other conditions.
- **Broccoli**
- **Main Benefit:** Packed with sulforaphane, an antioxidant that fights inflammation by reducing your levels of cytokines and NF-kB, which drive inflammation.
- **Avocados**

- **Main Benefit:** Loaded with potassium, magnesium, fiber, and heart-healthy monounsaturated fats, avocados offer anti-inflammatory benefits.
- **Green Tea**
- **Main Benefit:** Contains epigallocatechin gallate (EGCG), an antioxidant known to fight inflammation and reduce damage to the fatty acids in your cells.
- **Peppers (Bell Peppers and Chili Peppers)**
- **Main Benefit:** High in antioxidants and vitamin C, peppers have anti-inflammatory benefits and can also reduce oxidative stress.
- **Mushrooms (Portobello, Shiitake, Truffles)**
- **Main Benefit:** Low in calories and rich in selenium, copper, and all of the B vitamins, mushrooms have compounds that provide anti-inflammatory protection.
- **Grapes**
- **Main Benefit:** Contains anthocyanins, which reduce inflammation and may also reduce the risk of several diseases, including heart disease.
- **Turmeric**
- **Main Benefit:** The active ingredient, curcumin, has potent anti-inflammatory properties and is particularly effective in reducing inflammation in arthritis patients.
- **Extra Virgin Olive Oil**
- **Main Benefit:** Rich in monounsaturated fats and oleocanthal, it has similar anti-inflammatory effects to ibuprofen, reducing the risk of chronic diseases.
- **Dark Chocolate and Cocoa**
- **Main Benefit:** Flavanols in dark chocolate can reduce inflammation and may lower the risk of disease, acting as antioxidants.
- **Tomatoes**
- **Main Benefit:** High in lycopene, which reduces inflammation and can also help reduce the risk of several cancers.
- **Cherries**

- **Main Benefit:** Contains high levels of antioxidants, such as anthocyanins and catechins, which fight inflammation.
- **Nuts (Almonds, Walnuts)**
- **Main Benefit:** A great source of fiber, magnesium, vitamin E, and omega-3 fatty acids, nuts have anti-inflammatory properties that benefit heart health.
- **Ginger**
- **Main Benefit:** Gingerol, the main bioactive compound in ginger, has strong anti-inflammatory and antioxidant effects.
- **Leafy Greens (Spinach, Kale, Swiss Chard)**
- **Main Benefit:** High in antioxidants, vitamins, and minerals, leafy greens can reduce inflammation and protect against chronic diseases.

Meal Planning and Preparation Tips

Creating a meal plan doesn't have to feel like choreographing a complex Pilates sequence. Here's how to make it manageable and effective:

- **Plan:** Spend some time each week mapping out your meals. This prevents last-minute unhealthy choices and reduces stress.
- **Batch Cooking:** Prepare portions of proteins, grains, and veggies at the start of the week. Mix and match these for quick, balanced meals.
- **Snack Smart:** Eat healthy snacks for hunger strikes between meals. Greek yogurt, fruit, and raw nuts are great options.

In weaving nutrition into the fabric of your Pilates lifestyle, you're fueling your body and enriching your practice from the inside out. It's about creating harmony between movement and nourishment, allowing each to support and enhance the other. With each mindful bite and every purposeful movement, you're tending to your wellness garden, cultivating a state of health that's flourishing and vibrant.

WEEKLY MEAL PLAN

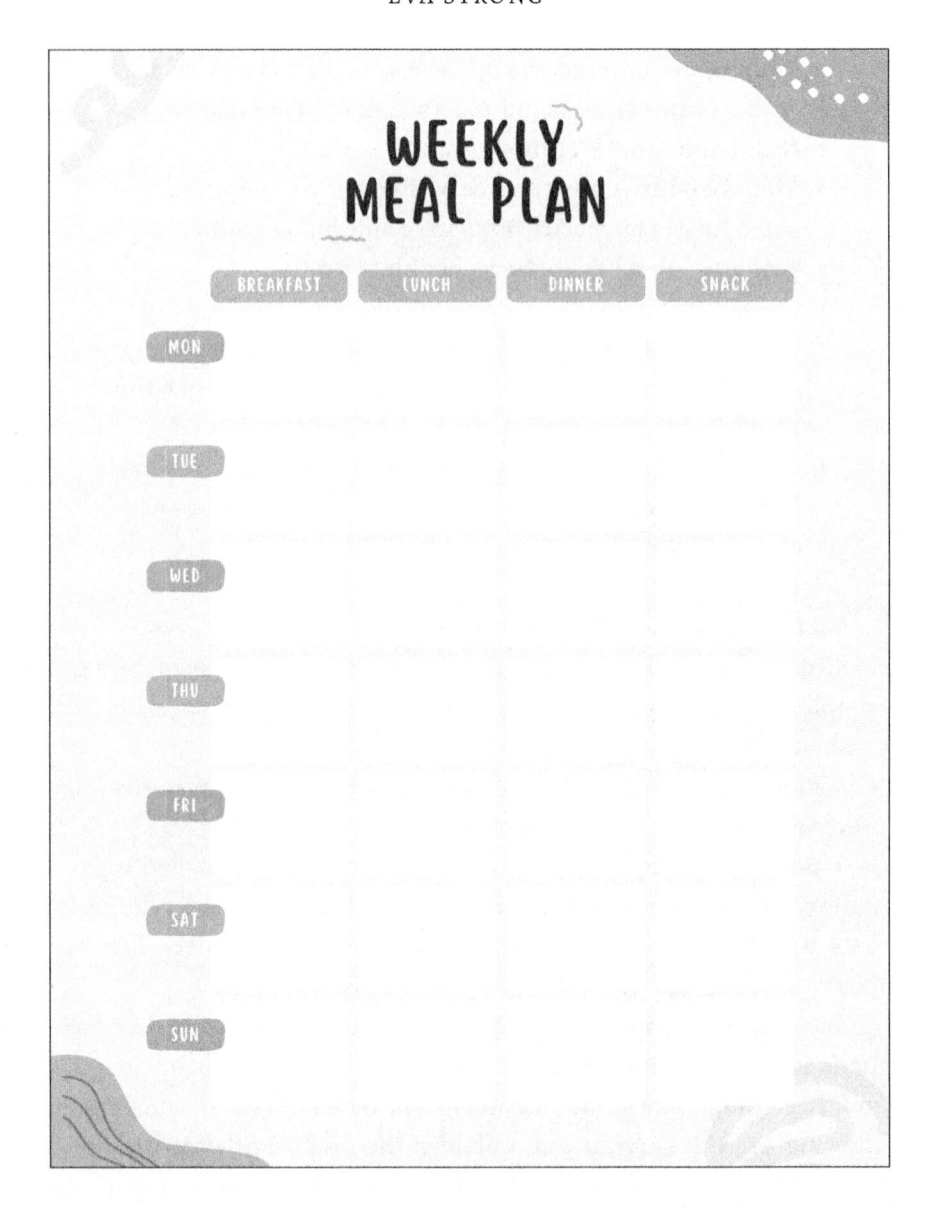

	BREAKFAST	LUNCH	DINNER	SNACK
MON				
TUE				
WED				
THU				
FRI				
SAT				
SUN				

5.1 THE IMPACT OF PILATES ON SLEEP AND RELAXATION

Sleep serves as the body's method of resetting, like hitting the refresh button on your browser, clearing away the day's stress, and preparing you for the challenges ahead. For many, especially seniors, achieving restful sleep can feel elusive. Here, we explore how incorporating Pilates into your routine can significantly enhance the quality of your slumber, drawing a direct line between the physical exertion of Pilates and the mental calm it induces, setting the stage for a night of deep, restorative sleep.

Pilates for Better Sleep

Pilates' gentle, controlled movements do more than improve your physical well-being; they're also incredibly effective at easing the mind. The focused nature of Pilates exercises, which demand mindfulness and deep breathing, naturally transitions the body into a state of relaxation. For seniors, this can be particularly beneficial. Physical activity helps to expend energy in a productive, stress-relieving way, ensuring that by bedtime, the body is in a more restful state, ready to embrace sleep. Moreover, the stress reduction associated with regular Pilates practice has been shown to decrease cortisol levels, the "stress hormone," further facilitating a peaceful night's sleep.

Relaxation Techniques Post-Pilates

After a Pilates session, implementing specific relaxation techniques can amplify the sleep-promoting effects of the workout. Here are a few to consider:

• **Guided Relaxation**: Lying down comfortably, perform a guided body scan, progressively relaxing each body part from head to toe.

• **Deep Breathing Exercises**: Practice deep, slow breathing techniques such as the 4-7-8 method, which involves inhaling for four seconds, holding the breath for seven seconds, and exhaling for eight seconds. This technique is known to reduce anxiety and prepare the body for sleep.

• **Gentle Stretching**: Engage in a series of light stretches, focusing on areas that tend to hold tension, like the neck, shoulders, and lower back. These stretches can further loosen the muscles and enhance the feeling of relaxation.

Creating a Pre-Sleep Pilates Routine

A short Pilates routine before bed can be the perfect segue into a night of deep, restorative sleep. This routine should focus on gentle stretches and calming breathwork rather than vigorous exercises to avoid stimulating the body too much before sleep. Consider incorporating movements such as:

- **Pelvic Tilts**: To gently engage and relax the lower back.
- **Spine Stretch**: Sitting with legs extended, reach forward slowly, focusing on breathing deeply to stretch the back and hamstrings.
- **Child's Pose**: A comforting pose that relieves back, neck, and shoulder tension.

Performing these exercises in a quiet, dimly lit space can enhance the calming effect, preparing both mind and body for sleep.

The Connection Between Mindful Movement and Sleep

The principle of mindfulness, a cornerstone of Pilates, emphasizes being present in the moment, a practice that can significantly impact mental relaxation and, by extension, sleep quality. The mindful movement practiced in Pilates—paying attention to breath, form, and the sensations of each movement—can help quiet the mind, steering it away from the day's worries and towards a calm readiness for sleep. This mindfulness does not just end with the practice; it extends into how you prepare for sleep, encouraging routines that support rather than disrupt sleep readiness, such as limiting screen time and engaging in calming activities before bed.

Integrating Pilates into your lifestyle does more than enhance physical fitness; it offers a holistic approach to well-being, encompassing the body and mind. Through the practices outlined above, Pilates emerges as a form of exercise and a comprehensive strategy for improving sleep quality and overall relaxation, particularly for seniors. By fostering a balance between exertion and relaxation, Pilates paves the way for nights of restful sleep, ensuring you wake up refreshed and ready to embrace the day with vitality and a clear mind.

5.2 BUILDING A COMMUNITY THROUGH PILATES

The magic of Pilates doesn't only unfold on the mat; it extends far beyond into the connections we forge with those around us. At its core, Pilates is about balance, strength, and community. This last aspect is often overlooked, yet it's as integral to your growth as the exercises themselves. Imagine a space where motivation flows freely, where every achievement is celebrated, and every setback is met with support. This is the power of community in Pilates. It's not just about sharing a space; it's about sharing a part of your journey, learning from each other, and growing together.

The Importance of Community in a Pilates Lifestyle

The path to maintaining an active lifestyle, especially in later years, can sometimes feel solitary. However, integrating into a Pilates community can significantly shift this perception. The encouragement in a community setting fosters a sense of belonging and purpose, making the practice more enjoyable and rewarding. It introduces an element of accountability, gently nudging you to stay committed even on days when motivation wanes. Additionally, it provides a platform for exchanging knowledge, where tips, experiences, and personal insights into Pilates become valuable shared resources.

Ways to Connect with the Pilates Community

- **Local Pilates Studios and Clubs:** These are great starting points. Many offer special classes geared towards seniors or beginner levels, providing a comfortable entry into the community. Look out for social events or workshops these studios host to further engage with fellow Pilates enthusiasts.

- **Online Forums and Social Media Groups:** The digital age brings the Pilates community to your fingertips. Joining online groups dedicated to Pilates offers a broader perspective, connecting you with practitioners from around the globe. These platforms are ripe with discussions, advice, and personal stories that can inspire and guide you.

- **Pilates Events and Retreats:** Attending these gatherings can be a transformative experience. They offer immersive learning opportunities and the chance to deepen connections within the Pilates community. Keep an eye out for events that cater to a wide range of abilities, ensuring an inclusive environment.

Sharing Pilates with Family and Friends

Introducing Pilates to your close circle can be incredibly rewarding. It's a chance to share something you're passionate about while encouraging a healthier lifestyle among those you care about. Here are some ways to get started:

- **Host a Pilates Day:** Invite family and friends for a casual Pilates session. Keep it light and fun, focusing on basic exercises everyone can try. It's a great way to introduce the practice in a relaxed setting.
- **Gift Pilates Classes:** Offering classes as a gift can be a thoughtful way to encourage loved ones to try Pilates. It might just be the nudge they need to start their journey.
- **Share Your Story:** Sometimes, all it takes is hearing about your positive experiences with Pilates. Share how it has impacted your life, the benefits you've noticed, and the enjoyment it brings. Your enthusiasm can be contagious.

Volunteering and Giving Back Through Pilates

Pilates is a gift that keeps giving, and sharing it with the community can be a profound way to give back. Here are some ideas:

- **Free Community Classes:** If you're an experienced practitioner or a certified instructor, consider offering free classes in local community centers. This can be especially impactful for those who might not have access to regular Pilates classes.
- **Pilates for a Cause:** Organize a Pilates event or class where the proceeds go to a local charity. It's a wonderful way to combine your love for Pilates with support for a good cause.
- **Volunteer at Senior Centers:** Many senior centers seek activities promoting an active lifestyle. Volunteering to lead a Pilates session can introduce seniors to the practice, offering them a new avenue for improving their health and well-being.

Building a community through Pilates enriches your practice in ways that go beyond the physical. It creates a network of support, motivation, and shared joy. This community becomes a part of your Pilates lifestyle, where every member, from the novice to the experienced practitioner, plays a crucial role. You celebrate the milestones together, work through the challenges, and appreciate the journey. Through these connections, Pilates becomes more than a series of exercises; it evolves into a shared experience that nurtures both body and soul.

5.3 PILATES AS A CATALYST FOR LIFESTYLE CHANGE

Pilates does more than sculpt your body and improve your posture; it reaches into every aspect of your life, encouraging transformations that extend well beyond the mat. This holistic approach to wellness can motivate shifts in diet, mental health, and how you interact with the world and people around you.

Personal Growth Through Pilates

The discipline required in Pilates, focusing on the precision of each movement and breath, mirrors the attentiveness needed to cultivate positive changes in your daily life. It's not just about physical flexibility but also gracefully adapting to life's challenges. Regular practice instills a sense of calm and resilience, invaluable traits as you navigate modern life's complexities. Moreover, the introspection encouraged by Pilates can lead to a deeper understanding of your body's needs, fostering a more nurturing approach to self-care and, by extension, how you care for others.

Setting and Achieving Lifestyle Goals

Pilates teaches the importance of setting intentions, whether perfecting a pose or enhancing your core strength. This principle is equally effective when applied to broader lifestyle goals. Here's a structured approach to setting and achieving these objectives, inspired by Pilates principles:

- **Define Clear, Achievable Goals:** Start with specific, measurable, and realistic goals. If stress reduction is your aim, define what that looks like. Perhaps it's dedicating 15 minutes daily to meditation or ensuring you get 7 hours of sleep each night.
- **Break Down Your Goals:** Just as Pilates movements are broken down into manageable parts, divide your goals into smaller, actionable steps. This could involve scheduling weekly meal prep time if your goal is to eat healthier or setting aside time daily for mindfulness practices.
- **Track Your Progress:** Keep a journal of your efforts and achieve-

ments. Reflecting on your progress can be incredibly motivating, like seeing your Pilates practice improve over time.

- **Be Patient and Persistent:** Remember, changes take time. Just as mastering a Pilates routine doesn't happen overnight, lifestyle transformations require patience and continuous effort.

Overcoming Obstacles with a Pilates Mindset

Every Pilates practitioner knows the journey includes moments of frustration and challenge. The same is true for lifestyle changes. Here are a few strategies inspired by Pilates to help overcome these hurdles:

- **Embrace Flexibility:** Just as Pilates requires adapting to what your body can do on any given day, approach your goals flexibly. If you miss a day of meditation, for example, don't dwell on it. Recognize the slip and refocus on your objective.
- **Maintain Focus:** Pilates demands concentration on your breath and movement. Apply this focused approach to your goals, keeping your end objective in sight and not allowing distractions to derail your efforts.
- **Celebrate Small Victories:** In Pilates, every small improvement is a step toward greater strength and flexibility. Celebrate the small wins in your lifestyle changes as well. Acknowledge a week of healthy eating or recognizing when you need a mental break as progress.

Success Stories of Transformation

Hearing about others who have transformed their lives through Pilates can be incredibly inspiring. Here are brief accounts of individuals who found Pilates the catalyst for wider change:

- **Mia:** After starting Pilates to improve her posture, Mia noticed significantly decreased stress levels. This newfound calm encouraged her to explore meditation, leading to a more mindful approach to life. Pilates was the first step in a comprehensive journey toward mental and emotional well-being.
- **Carlos:** Carlos turned to Pilates as part of his rehabilitation from a knee injury. The focus on low-impact exercises accelerated his recovery and inspired a lifestyle overhaul. He adopted a healthier diet to support his physical healing, ultimately losing weight and feeling more energized than in years. For Carlos, Pilates was the gateway to a revitalized life.

- **Ellen:** Finding Pilates in her 60s, Ellen was amazed by the boost in her energy and improved sleep quality. Motivated by these changes, she began volunteering in her community, something she hadn't felt the confidence or energy to do before. Pilates ignited a sense of purpose and community engagement that enriched Ellen's life profoundly.

These stories underscore the holistic impact of Pilates. It's an exercise regimen and a lifestyle philosophy that encourages growth, resilience, and a deep connection with oneself and the community. As you continue your Pilates practice, let it guide you in achieving physical strength and flexibility and nurturing a lifestyle that reflects your highest health, happiness, and well-being aspirations.

5.4 THE LEGACY OF PILATES IN SENIOR WELLNESS: LOOKING FORWARD

Pilates stands as a beacon of hope and resilience, especially for those in their golden years. Its imprint on senior health and wellness is profound, offering more than just physical benefits. This practice is a testament to the idea that age should never be a barrier to improving one's quality of life. It's a tool that fosters longevity, nurtures independence, and enriches the overall journey of aging.

Pilates isn't merely a series of exercises to be performed; it's a philosophy to be lived. It adapts as you do, gracefully meeting you at every stage of your aging process. This adaptability ensures that Pilates can be a constant companion throughout life, evolving to address changing health and fitness needs. Pilates respects the body's wisdom at every age, from modifications for those just starting their fitness journey to challenges for the seasoned practitioner.

The beauty of Pilates is that it creates ripples beyond the individual, influencing families and communities to embrace a culture of wellness. Sharing the practice and its myriad benefits catalyzes a larger movement toward health and vitality. It's not just about personal gain but about uplifting those around you, contributing to a legacy of wellness that transcends generations. This shared experience fosters a sense of communal well-being, making the journey towards health a collective endeavor.

Looking ahead, the horizon of Pilates for seniors is vibrant with potential. Research continuously unveils new insights into how Pilates can be tailored to better serve the aging population. Innovations in teaching methods, integration with technology, and fusion with other wellness practices are expanding the scope of Pilates. These advancements promise a future where Pilates remains at the forefront of senior wellness, adaptable, and relevant in addressing the multifaceted needs of aging bodies.

As we peer into the future, it's clear that Pilates for seniors is more than just a trend; it's a growing field ripe with opportunity. The emphasis on low-impact movements, core strength, and flexibility aligns perfectly with the needs of aging bodies, making Pilates an ideal practice for maintaining mobility and independence. With the promise of new research and developments, Pilates is poised to continue evolving, offering even more ways to support senior health and wellness in the years to come.

This vision of Pilates as a lifelong practice is not just about maintaining physical health; it's about nurturing a sense of vitality, connection, and joy well into our later years. It encourages us to look forward with optimism, embracing the changes that come with aging as opportunities for growth and discovery. As we continue to share and evolve the practice of Pilates, we contribute to a culture that values and supports aging with dignity, strength, and grace.

In this light, Pilates becomes more than exercise; it's a pathway to a life well-lived, marked by an unwavering commitment to personal and communal well-being. It's a promise that we can continue to grow, learn, and thrive regardless of age. This legacy of wellness, grounded in the principles of Pilates, offers a powerful blueprint for senior health—a vision that we carry forward together into the future.

As the chapters of our lives unfold, let us carry the essence of Pilates with us—a practice that strengthens our bodies and enriches our souls. Let this be a reminder that in Pilates, as in life, there is always room for growth, connection, and renewal.

6

BEGINNERS WALL PILATES 10-MINUTE ROUTINE

Here's a gentle and accessible 10-minute weekly wall Pilates routine designed specifically for seniors at a beginner level. This routine focuses on improving balance, flexibility, and strength while ensuring safety and comfort.

Note: Before beginning any new exercise program, seniors should consult a healthcare provider.

DAY 1: INTRODUCTION TO WALL PILATES

1. Wall Roll Down (2 minutes):

- Begin by standing with your back flush against the wall. Keep your feet hip-width apart and planted firmly on the ground.
- Take a deep breath, and as you exhale, start tucking your chin towards your chest and slowly rolling your spine down the wall.
- Bend your knees as you roll down, allowing your back to slide down the wall smoothly.
- Go down as far as comfortable, then with a deep inhale, reverse the motion, unrolling your spine up the wall to return to the starting position.
- Repeat this roll-down and roll-up motion smoothly for 2 minutes.

2. Wall Push-ups (2 minutes):

- Face the wall and stand slightly more than arm's length away, placing your hands flat against the wall at shoulder height and width.
- Step your feet back slightly so you're leaning into the wall at an angle.
- Inhale as you bend your elbows and lower your chest towards the wall, maintaining a straight line with your body.
- Exhale as you push yourself back to the starting position.
- Perform this push-up motion for 2 minutes, maintaining a solid core and not letting your hips sag.

3. Wall Squats (2 minutes):

- Stand with your back against the wall, feet hip-width apart and about two feet from the wall.

- Slide your back down the wall as you bend your knees, entering a squat position. Aim to get your thighs parallel to the floor.
- Hold this squat position for a few seconds, keeping the weight in your heels.
- Press down through your heels to slide back up the wall to the starting position.
- Continue this movement for 2 minutes, using the wall to help you maintain balance.

4. Standing Toe Raises (2 minutes):

- Face the wall, standing arm's length away, and place your hands on the wall for balance.
- Keep your feet hip-width apart and flat on the ground.
- Slowly raise your heels as high as possible, coming onto your toes while keeping the balls of your feet on the ground.
- Lower your heels back down with control.
- Repeat this calf-raising motion for 2 minutes, feeling the stretch and contraction in your calf muscles.

5. Deep Breathing (2 minutes):

- Stand with your back against the wall, feet hip-width apart, and hands relaxed by your sides or on your abdomen.
- Close your eyes to help focus your mind inward.
- Inhale deeply through your nose, expanding your ribcage and filling your lungs with air.
- Hold your breath for a moment at the peak of your inhalation.
- Exhale slowly through your mouth or nose, contracting your abdominal muscles to empty all the air.
- Continue this deep, conscious breathing pattern for 2 minutes, allowing your body to relax more with each breath.

This routine focuses on controlled movements and breath, aiming to build strength and stability while promoting relaxation and mindfulness.

GENTLE WALL PILATES FOR SENIORS:

DAY 2: CORE AND LEGS

1. Wall Plank (2 minutes):

- Stand facing the wall at an arm's length away.
- Lean forward and place your hands on the wall at shoulder height, keeping your arms straight.
- Walk your feet back until your body is straight from head to heels as if you're about to do a push-up against the wall.
- Engage your core muscles, tuck your pelvis slightly, and keep your body rigid.
- Hold this plank position for 2 minutes, focusing on form and steady breathing.

2. Leg Slides (2 minutes):

- For balance, stand with one side of your body near the wall, lightly touching the wall with one hand.
- Place your weight on the leg closest to the wall.
- Slowly slide the other leg out to the side, keeping it straight and the foot flexed.
- Glide the leg back to the starting position.
- You should continue smoothly sliding the leg in and out for 1 minute before switching to the other side for the remaining minute.

3. Wall Slides (2 minutes):

- Stand with your back flat against the wall, feet about hip-width apart and slightly away from the wall.
- Raise your arms over your head, engaging your core.
- Slowly slide your arms down bending your elbows until they are at a bend of 90 degrees, trying to keep your wrists, elbows, and arms in contact with the wall.
- Slide your arms back up to the starting position.

- Repeat this motion for 2 minutes, working on shoulder mobility and engagement of the upper back muscles.

4. Standing Knee Lifts (2 minutes):

- Stand with your back against the wall for support.
- Keep your feet hip-width apart and arms by your sides or resting on your hips.
- Slowly lift one knee towards your chest while keeping the standing leg straight.
- Lower the knee back down in a controlled movement.
- Alternate legs after each lift, performing this exercise for 2 minutes.

5. Relaxation (2 minutes):

- Finish the routine by standing with your back against the wall.
- Let your arms hang loosely at your sides, or place them gently on your abdomen.
- Close your eyes, and take deep breaths through your nose, filling your lungs fully.
- Exhale slowly through your mouth or nose, feeling your body relax and releasing tension with each breath.
- Continue deep breathing for 2 minutes, allowing your mind and body to enter a state of relaxation.

GENTLE WALL PILATES FOR SENIORS:

DAY 3: FLEXIBILITY AND BALANCE

1. Wall Arm Circles (2 minutes):

- Stand with one side of your body facing the wall, about an arm's length away.
- Extend the arm closest to the wall out to the side, palm facing down.
- Begin making small circles with the extended arm. Make sure the circles are controlled and the movement comes from the shoulder joint.
- After one minute, turn around so the other side of your body is next to the wall, and repeat with the other arm.

2. Wall Hip Circles (2 minutes):

- Stand facing the wall with your hands resting on the wall for support.
- Shift your weight to one leg and lift the other off the ground.
- Start making gentle circles with the raised leg, moving from the hip. Keep the movements smooth and controlled.
- After one minute, switch to the other leg and repeat the hip circles.

3. Pelvic Tilts (2 minutes):

- Stand with your back against the wall, feet hip-width apart, and knees slightly bent.
- Press the small of your back into the wall and tilt your pelvis forward, tightening the abdominal muscles.
- Then, arch your back slightly off the wall, tilting the pelvis back.
- Continue tilting your pelvis forward and back, maintaining a slow and controlled movement.

4. Wall Torso Twists (2 minutes):

- Stand with one side of your body next to the wall, feet planted firmly and hip-width apart.
- Press your hand against the wall at chest height for light support.
- Keep your hips facing forward and gently twist your upper body towards the wall.
- Return to the starting position and repeat the twisting motion.
- After one minute, switch sides so the other side of your body is next to the wall and continue the torso twists.

5. Cool Down Stretch (2 minutes):

- Stand with your back against the wall and your feet hip-width apart.
- Reach your arms overhead, with the back of your hands against the wall, and gently press your arms back to stretch your chest and shoulders.
- Hold the position for a stretch that feels comfortable, breathing deeply and focusing on relaxing any areas of tension.
- To stretch your back, place your hands on the wall at waist height and step back until your body is at a 90-degree angle, similar to a downward-facing dog position in yoga. Gently press your chest toward the floor to deepen the stretch.
- Hold each stretch for several deep breaths before releasing.

Remember to breathe naturally throughout the exercises and make smooth, controlled movements. The focus should be on feeling a gentle stretch and engagement of the muscles without any strain.

GENTLE WALL PILATES FOR SENIORS:

DAY 4: UPPER BODY AND POSTURE

1. Wall Prayer Stretch (2 minutes):

- Stand with your back flat against the wall, feet shoulder-width apart.
- Bring your palms together in front of you at chest level in a prayer position, with your elbows out to the sides.
- Press your palms firmly together, engaging your chest muscles.
- While keeping your hands pressed, gently squeeze your shoulder blades toward the wall, activating the muscles in your upper back.
- Hold the squeeze for a few seconds, then release slightly without separating your palms or elbows.
- Repeat this squeezing and releasing motion for 2 minutes, maintaining the integrity of the posture.

2. Wall Bicep Curls (2 minutes):

- Stand facing away from the wall with your back close to it.
- Press your elbows back into the wall at about waist height.
- Raise your hands toward your shoulders in a bicep curl motion, as if holding weights with your palms facing up or toward each other.
- Extend your arms back down, straightening them fully while keeping your elbows in contact with the wall.
- Continue the bicep curl motion for 2 minutes, keeping your movements slow and controlled.

3. Shoulder Blade Squeeze (2 minutes):

- Stand with your back against the wall and arms relaxed by your sides.
- Squeeze your shoulder blades together, drawing them toward the wall and down your back.

- As you squeeze, allow your arms to naturally move back slightly, opening up your chest.
- Hold the squeeze for a few seconds, then release slowly.
- Repeat this motion for 2 minutes, focusing on the movement between the shoulder blades.

4. Chest Opener (2 minutes):

- Stand facing away from the wall with your feet a step away from it.
- Extend your arms out to the sides and place your palms on the wall at shoulder height.
- Gently lean your torso forward without bending at the hips, opening up the chest.
- You should feel a stretch across your chest and front shoulders.
- Hold the stretch for a few seconds, then return to the starting position.
- Repeat the movement for 2 minutes, taking care not to overstretch.

5. Neck and Shoulder Relaxation (2 minutes):

- Stand with your back to the wall, with your feet shoulder-width apart.
- Gently roll your head from one shoulder to another, keeping the movements slow and mindful to avoid strain.
- After rolling your head a few times, move on to shoulder rolls.
- Roll your shoulders up toward your ears, then back, pressing your shoulder blades down together and finally releasing them forward.
- Continue this circular motion for the remainder of the 2 minutes, letting go of any tension in your neck and shoulders with each roll.

Throughout this routine, keep your spine aligned against the wall and move smoothly to prevent jerky movements or unnecessary pressure, particularly in the neck and shoulder areas. The focus should be on stretching and strengthening with control; synchronization with your breath will enhance relaxation.

DAY 5: CORE ENGAGEMENT AND STABILITY

1. Wall Dead Bug (2 minutes):

- Lie on the floor with your legs up, your feet flat against the wall, and your hips and knees bent at a 90-degree angle.
- Press your lower back into the floor to engage your core.
- Slowly extend one leg out, straightening the knee to slide your foot down the wall while the other remains in place.
- Return the extended leg to the starting position.
- Alternate extending each leg, maintaining core engagement, and pressing your lower back to the floor.
- Continue alternating for 2 minutes.

2. Wall Side Leg Lifts (2 minutes):

- Stand with one side of your body close to the wall for support.
- Place the hand closest to the wall on the wall for balance.
- Lift the leg farther from the wall sideways away from your body, keeping it straight and your torso upright.
- Lower the leg back down with control.
- After 1 minute, turn around so the other side of your body is next to the wall, and repeat the leg lifts with the other leg for another minute.

3. Standing Pelvic Tilts (2 minutes):

- Stand with your back against the wall, your feet shoulder-width apart, and your knees slightly bent.
- Press your lower back into the wall to flatten it, engaging your abdominal muscles.
- Then, arch your lower back slightly, creating a small space between your lower back and the wall.
- Repeat these pelvic tilts, arching and flattening your lower back against the wall.

- Continue for 2 minutes, maintaining a smooth and controlled motion.

4. Wall Sit (2 minutes):

- Stand with your back against the wall, feet shoulder-width apart and about 2 feet from the wall.
- Slide down the wall into a seated position, with your thighs parallel to the floor and knees over your ankles.
- Hold this position for 2 minutes, engaging your core and ensuring your back is flat against the wall.
- Keep your arms either by your sides or in front of you for added stability.

5. Tailbone Presses (2 minutes):

- Sit with your back against the wall, knees bent, and feet flat on the ground about hip-width apart.
- Focus on your tailbone and use your lower abdominal muscles to press your tailbone towards the floor.
- You should feel your lower abdominals engaging without using your legs or glutes to press down.
- Hold the engagement for a few seconds, then release it slightly.
- Repeat these tailbone presses for 2 minutes, keeping your movements slow and controlled.

For all exercises, focus on maintaining proper form and controlled movements. Remember to breathe consistently throughout each movement, and only perform movements within your comfortable range to avoid strain.

DAY 6: BALANCE AND COORDINATION

1. Single Leg Wall Press (2 minutes):

- Stand about an arm's length facing the wall.
- Press one hand against the wall for support and slowly lift the opposite leg, keeping it straight or slightly bending the knee for balance.
- Engage your core to maintain balance and stand tall through your supporting leg.
- Hold this position for one minute, focusing on stability.
- After one minute, switch to press the other hand against the wall and lift the opposite leg.
- Continue to engage your core and focus on your balance for the second minute.

2. Wall Bird Dog (2 minutes):

- Stand a few feet away from the wall, your feet hip-width apart.
- Lean forward from the hips and place your hands flat on the wall at shoulder height.
- Engage your core and extend one arm as if reaching above your head.
- At the same time, extend the opposite leg straight back, keeping your foot flexed.
- Hold this extended position for a few seconds, maintaining a straight line from your fingers to your toes and keeping your hips square to the wall.
- Carefully bring your arm and leg back to the starting position.
- Repeat the movement with the opposite arm and leg.
- Continue alternating sides for 2 minutes, ensuring each movement is deliberate and controlled.

3. Heel Raises (2 minutes):

- Stand with your back flat against the wall, feet hip-width apart.
- Slowly raise your heels off the ground, pressing up onto the balls of your feet.
- Keep your body straight, with your shoulders and back against the wall.
- Lower your heels back to the floor with control.
- Repeat the heel raises for 2 minutes, focusing on maintaining balance and engaging your calf muscles.

4. **Wall Warrior Pose (2 minutes):**

- Face the wall in a staggered stance, with your front foot pointing forward and your back foot positioned at about a 45-degree angle.
- Extend your arms overhead, with your hands flat against the wall.
- Bend your front knee, ensure it stays over the ankle, and press into the wall as if trying to push it away.
- Keep your back leg straight and heel grounded.
- Maintain the warrior pose for 2 minutes, engaging your core and quads for balance and stability.

5. **Wall-assisted Leg Swings (2 minutes):**

- Stand side-on to the wall, lightly holding it with one hand for support.
- Shift your weight to the leg closest to the wall.
- Swing the outside leg forward and back in a controlled motion, keeping your torso stable.
- Allow your hip to open up with the forward swing and stretch out on the backward swing.
- After 1 minute, switch sides and repeat the leg swings with the other leg.

Remember to keep your movements smooth and your breathing

even throughout the routine. Engage your core muscles for stability, and do not rush through the motions. Focus on form and control to maximize the benefits of each exercise.

DAY 7: GENTLE STRETCH AND RELAXATION

1. Wall-assisted Hamstring Stretch (2 minutes):

- Sit on the floor facing the wall with your legs extended straight in front of you and your heels pressed against the wall.
- Keep your back straight, and your toes pointed upwards.
- Slowly reach forward with your hands towards your toes, hinging at your hips, not rounding your back. You should feel a stretch along the back of your legs.
- Hold the position gently, breathing deeply and gradually, allowing the stretch to deepen.
- Maintain this stretch for 2 minutes, focusing on relaxing into the stretch without forcing your toes.

2. Arm and Shoulder Stretch (2 minutes):

- Stand facing the wall at an arm's length distance.
- Extend your arms forward and place your palms flat against the wall at shoulder height.
- Gently lean your body forward, allowing your chest to move towards the wall while keeping your heels on the ground.
- You should feel a stretch through your shoulders, chest, and arms.
- Hold this position for 2 minutes, breathing deeply and gently, increasing the stretch.

3. Wall-assisted Calf Stretch (2 minutes):

- Face the wall and stand about an arm's length away.
- Step one foot back, keeping that heel pressed to the floor and the front knee slightly bent.
- Lean into the wall, keeping your back leg straight to feel a stretch in the calf of the back leg.

- Hold the stretch for 1 minute, then switch legs and repeat for another minute.
- Ensure your back heel remains pressed to the floor to maintain the stretch.

4. Wall-assisted Spinal Twist (2 minutes):

- Sit on the floor with one side of your body against the wall.
- Extend your legs in front of you, then gently twist your torso towards the wall.
- Use your arms for gentle support, not to force the twist.
- Hold the twist for 1 minute, breathing deeply and allowing your spine to lengthen and rotate gently.
- Switch sides and repeat the twist for another minute, focusing on maintaining a gentle, even stretch throughout the twist.

5. Deep Breathing and Relaxation (2 minutes):

- Finish the routine by sitting or standing with your back against the wall.
- Close your eyes and focus on taking slow, deep breaths.
- Inhale deeply through your nose, filling your lungs, then exhale slowly through your mouth or nose.
- With each exhale, focus on releasing any remaining tension in your body.
- Continue this focused deep breathing for 2 minutes, allowing yourself to relax fully.

Throughout each stretch, focus on gentle, controlled breathing and avoid pushing into pain. The goal is to feel a soft stretch and release tension, not to force flexibility.

THIS WEEKLY 10-MINUTE ROUTINE IS DESIGNED TO BE ACCESSIBLE AND beneficial for seniors, focusing on enhancing mobility, stability, and

GENTLE WALL PILATES FOR SENIORS:

overall well-being through gentle and effective wall Pilates exercises.

CONCLUSION

Phew, what a ride, right? From the very first page, we've journeyed together through the world of Pilates, exploring its incredible power to transform our bodies and enrich our golden years with strength, flexibility, and vitality. We've delved deep into the core of Pilates, navigating through its principles and unveiling exercises that are as beneficial as they are enjoyable. Together, we've sketched out how to weave Pilates into the very fabric of our daily lives, tackled advanced techniques, and illuminated the holistic impact embracing a Pilates lifestyle can have.

The essence of our adventure? Pilates isn't just about stretching or holding poses; it's a beacon guiding us toward a more vibrant, fulfilling aging process. It's the key to unlocking a physically more robust version of ourselves, sure, but also a more mentally resilient and socially connected one.

If there's anything I want you to walk away with, it's this: the transformative power of Pilates for seniors is real. It's profound. It's not merely about keeping fit; it's about rewriting the narrative of aging into one of continued growth and discovery. I've seen it firsthand, not only in my practice but in the lives of countless seniors who've found a renewed zest for life in Pilates.

CONCLUSION

So, what's next? The ball's in your court. With all the enthusiasm I can muster, I urge you to keep this momentum going. Seek out classes, find your community, challenge yourself with new poses, and make Pilates a steadfast companion in your journey toward wellness. Remember, every day offers a unique chance to enhance your practice and, by extension, your life.

I want to share a little nugget from my own experience. There was a moment, some years back, when I witnessed the transformation of a dear friend who embraced Pilates in her senior years. Her journey from skepticism to seeing tangible changes in her posture, mood, and overall well-being was inspiring. It's stories like hers that fuel my passion and, I hope, ignite a spark in you too.

Thank you for allowing me to participate in your exploration of Pilates. I sincerely hope you've found inspiration, guidance, and perhaps a dash of excitement to pursue a path of wellness that resonates deeply with you. And remember, this is merely the beginning. Keep an eye out for more resources from me — whether it's a follow-up book, online materials, workshops, or community gatherings. Our journey together continues, and I can't wait to see where it takes us.

As we part ways (at least until you pick up another one of my resources), I leave you with a thought that encapsulates our shared journey:

"Physical fitness is the first requisite of happiness." – Joseph Pilates.

May you find happiness, health, and an unbridled sense of adventure on your Pilates journey. Here's to bending, stretching, and growing — in all ways, always.

With gratitude and warmth,

Eva Strong

FREQUENTLY ASKED QUESTIONS

These questions and answers aim to cover the broad and varied aspects of Wall Pilates for seniors, from health benefits and getting started to overcoming obstacles and integrating them into a more general fitness plan. This FAQ is a comprehensive guide for seniors interested in starting or enhancing their Wall Pilates practice.

1. What is Wall Pilates?

Wall Pilates is a form of Pilates exercise that uses a wall as support, making it ideal for seniors looking for a safe way to enhance flexibility, strength, and balance.

2. How does Wall Pilates benefit seniors?

It improves posture, reduces the risk of falls by enhancing balance, increases flexibility, strengthens core muscles, and supports overall mental well-being.

3. Can Wall Pilates help with arthritis?

Yes, it can help alleviate arthritis symptoms by improving joint mobility and reducing stiffness through gentle stretching and strengthening exercises.

4. Is Wall Pilates safe for osteoporosis?

Absolutely, but always consult with a healthcare provider first. Wall

Pilates can be modified to be safe for those with osteoporosis, focusing on improving bone density and reducing fall risk.

5. What equipment do I need?

No special equipment is needed, just a clear wall space. For some exercises, you may use a mat for comfort.

6. Can Wall Pilates improve my balance?

Yes, it explicitly targets balance improvement, reducing the likelihood of falls by enhancing your stability through core strengthening exercises.

7. How often should seniors practice Wall Pilates?

Two to three times a week is recommended, allowing for rest days between sessions.

8. Are there different levels of Wall Pilates exercises?

Yes, exercises can be adjusted for difficulty, from beginner to advanced, ensuring you progress comfortably.

9. Will Wall Pilates help with chronic back pain?

Many practitioners find relief from chronic back pain through Wall Pilates's core strengthening and posture-improving aspects.

10. Is Wall Pilates suitable for those who haven't exercised in a while?

Definitely. It's an excellent starting point for seniors looking to become more active, with modifications available to suit all fitness levels.

11. How does Wall Pilates compare to traditional Pilates?

Wall Pilates offers additional support and stability, making it more accessible for seniors or those with mobility issues without sacrificing the core principles of Pilates.

12. Can Wall Pilates help with weight management?

While not a high-intensity workout, it can contribute to weight management as part of an overall healthy lifestyle.

13. What if I have balance issues?

Wall Pilates is ideal for improving balance, with the wall providing the necessary support as you gain confidence in your stability.

14. Can Wall Pilates improve my posture?

Yes, it focuses on strengthening the core and back muscles, which are essential for good posture.

FREQUENTLY ASKED QUESTIONS

15. How quickly will I see results from Wall Pilates?

Individual results vary, but many notice posture, flexibility, and balance improvements within a few weeks of regular practice.

16. Are there any age restrictions for Wall Pilates?

No, Wall Pilates is beneficial and adaptable for seniors of all ages, focusing on individual capabilities.

17. Can Wall Pilates help with stress?

Yes, Pilates' mindful, focused movements can help reduce stress and improve mental clarity.

18. What should I wear for Wall Pilates?

Wear comfortable, non-restrictive clothing that allows for a full range of motion.

19. Do I need a Pilates instructor, or can I do it at home?

While an instructor can provide personalized guidance, many Wall Pilates exercises are simple enough to practice safely at home.

20. Can Wall Pilates improve my sleep?

Yes, the physical activity and stress reduction aspects of Wall Pilates can contribute to better sleep quality.

21. How do I start Wall Pilates as a complete beginner?

Begin with basic exercises focusing on breathing and gentle stretches. Gradually increase complexity as you become more comfortable.

22. Can Wall Pilates help me recover from surgery?

With the doctor's approval, it can be an excellent rehabilitation exercise, promoting gentle movement and strength rebuilding.

23. How long should a Wall Pilates session last for seniors?

A session can be as short as 20 minutes, but aim for 30 to 60 minutes for maximum benefit, depending on your fitness level.

24. Will Wall Pilates increase my flexibility?

Yes, regular practice stretches and lengthens the muscles, leading to improved flexibility over time.

25. Is there a risk of injury with Wall Pilates?

Wall Pilates is low-risk when performed correctly, especially with the wall providing stability and support.

26. How can I ensure I'm doing Wall Pilates correctly without an instructor?

Start with instructional videos or books tailored for seniors, focusing on proper form and gentle progression.

27. Can Wall Pilates help with knee pain?

Yes, by strengthening the muscles around the knees, it can help reduce pain and improve function.

28. What's the best time of day to practice Wall Pilates?

Anytime that fits your schedule is beneficial, though many find morning sessions energize them for the day ahead.

29. Can I do Wall Pilates if I have high blood pressure?

Consult with a healthcare provider, but many find the gentle nature of Wall Pilates suitable for managing high blood pressure.

30. How can Wall Pilates complement my existing workout routine?

It's an excellent addition to improving core strength, flexibility, and balance, enhancing overall fitness and performance.

31. Will I need to modify Wall Pilates exercises as I age?

Modifications can help you continue practicing safely and effectively, adapting to your body's changing needs.

32. Can Wall Pilates help with sciatica?

Strengthening the core and improving flexibility can alleviate sciatica symptoms for some individuals.

33. What are the mental health benefits of Wall Pilates?

It promotes mindfulness, reduces stress, and can improve cognitive function through focused movement and breathing.

34. Can Wall Pilates help improve my golf swing?

The core strength, flexibility, and balance gained can enhance your swing and overall performance.

35. How does Wall Pilates support heart health?

While not aerobic, its stress-reducing and blood pressure-lowering effects contribute to overall heart health.

36. Are there community groups or classes for senior Wall Pilates?

Many communities offer Pilates classes tailored to seniors, providing support and social interaction.

37. Can Wall Pilates be therapeutic for emotional well-being?

Its focus on mindfulness and body awareness can have therapeutic effects on emotional health.

38. What should I do if I experience pain during Wall Pilates?

Stop immediately and consult with a healthcare provider to ensure it's appropriate for you and to make necessary modifications.

39. How can I track my progress with Wall Pilates?

Keep a journal of your exercises, noting increased flexibility, balance improvements, and any changes in pain or well-being.

40. Can Wall Pilates help with digestion?

The movements can stimulate the digestive system, potentially improving digestion and alleviating bloating.

41. What if I don't feel any improvement?

Patience is vital. Physical and mental benefits can take time to manifest. Ensure your technique is correct, and consider consulting a Pilates instructor.

42. How does Wall Pilates help with aging?

It promotes an active lifestyle, supports mobility and independence, and contributes to a higher quality of life as we age.

43. Is Wall Pilates effective for weight loss?

While not a high-calorie burn exercise, it can support weight loss efforts by improving muscle tone and overall physical health.

44. Can I do Wall Pilates with a friend or partner?

Practicing with a friend can be motivating and enjoyable, making it easier to stick with your routine.

45. How does Wall Pilates compare to yoga?

Both focus on flexibility and mental wellness, but Wall Pilates emphasizes core strengthening and physical rehabilitation more.

46. Can Wall Pilates help with sleep issues?

Yes, Wall Pilates's relaxation and stress-relief benefits can contribute to better sleep quality for seniors.

47. How often should seniors practice Wall Pilates to see benefits?

Ideally, practicing 2-3 times a week can help seniors begin to notice improvements in strength, flexibility, and well-being.

48. Is Wall Pilates safe for those with osteoporosis?

With modifications and under the guidance of a healthcare

provider, Wall Pilates can be safe and beneficial for individuals with osteoporosis, focusing on bone health and fall prevention.

49. Can Wall Pilates exercises be done with a wheelchair?

Many Wall Pilates exercises can be adapted for individuals in wheelchairs, focusing on upper body strength and core stability.

50. How does Wall Pilates aid in managing chronic conditions like arthritis?

By enhancing joint mobility, reducing stiffness, and improving muscle strength, Wall Pilates can help manage arthritis symptoms and improve the quality of life for seniors.

KEEPING THE GAME ALIVE

Congratulations on reaching the end of this journey into Pilates! Now that you've got all the know-how to fold Pilates into your everyday routine, it's time to pass the torch and guide other readers to the same discoveries you've made.

Your thoughts and experiences with this book are invaluable, and by sharing your honest review on Amazon, you can point other seniors in the right direction. Imagine how your words could impact someone else's fitness and well-being journey!

Your contribution keeps the cycle of knowledge and passion for fitness going strong. With your help, we're not just sharing tips and tricks but building a community of health and vitality.

>>> Ready to share the love? [Scan here to leave your review on Amazon]

Thank you for being a vital part of our mission. You're not just practicing Pilates; you're inspiring it.

- With gratitude, Eva Strong

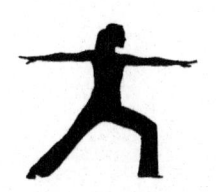

FITNESS TRACKER AND MONTHLY CALENDAR

FITNESS TRACKER AND MONTHLY CALENDAR

Daily fitness tracker

DATE:

M T W T F S S

DAILY GOALS: _____

NUTRITION TRACKER

Water	Breakfast	Lunch	Dinner	Snaks	Sweets & Desserts

WORKOUT PLAN / EXERCISE LOG

#	Exercise type	Sets	Reps	Intensity	✗/✓	Sets	Reps	Intensity
1.								
2.								
3.								
4.								
5.								
6.								
7.								
8.								
9.								
10.								
11.								
12.								
13.								
14.								
15.								

MOOD AND ENERGY LEVELS

REST AND RECOVERY

Time	Type

FITNESS TRACKER AND MONTHLY CALENDAR

MONTH: _____ YEAR: _____

SUNDAY	MONDAY	TUESDAY	WEDNESDAY	THURSDAY	FRIDAY	SATURDAY

NOTES	TO DO

REFERENCES

Adapting exercises while preserving the legacy of pilates. (n.d.). Human Kinetics. https://us.humankinetics.com/blogs/excerpt/adapting-exercises-while-preserving-the-legacy-of-pilates

Benefits of pilates in the elderly population: A systematic review and meta-analysis. (2022a). *European Journal of Investigation in Health, Psychology and Education, 12*(3). https://doi.org/10.3390/ejihpe12030018

Benefits of pilates in the elderly population: A systematic review and meta-analysis. (2022b). *European Journal of Investigation in Health, Psychology and Education, 12*(3). https://doi.org/10.3390/ejihpe12030018

Benefits of pilates in the elderly population: A systematic review and meta-analysis. (2022c). *European Journal of Investigation in Health, Psychology and Education, 12*(3). https://doi.org/10.3390/ejihpe12030018

Benefits of pilates in the elderly population: A systematic review and meta-analysis. (2022d). *European Journal of Investigation in Health, Psychology and Education, 12*(3). https://doi.org/10.3390/ejihpe12030018

Blyth, L. (2016, June 28). *Joseph pilates: The history & philosophy behind his exercise.* Flavours Holidays. https://www.flavoursholidays.co.uk/blog/joseph-pilates-history-philosophy/

Easy pilates prop alternatives you can find at home. (n.d.). Pilates Anytime. https://www.pilatesanytime.com/blog/equipment/pilates-prop-substitutions#:~:text=A%20blanket%20or%20large%20towel,but%20also%20fun%20and%20new

Effect of pilates on sleep quality: A systematic review and meta-analysis of randomized controlled trials. (2020). *Frontiers in Neurology, 11.* https://doi.org/10.3389/fneur.2020.00158

Effects of pilates training on physiological and psychological health parameters in healthy older adults and in older adults with clinical conditions over 55 years: A meta-analytical review. (2021). *Frontiers in Neurology, 12.* https://doi.org/10.3389/fneur.2021.724218

Guidelines to follow for eating during your pilates sessions. (n.d.). Verywell Fit. https://www.verywellfit.com/what-should-you-eat-for-doing-pilates-2704405

How to choose the best pilates app in 2024? (free & paid) » best software & apps — tested & reviewed for you. (2023, January 14). Today\'s Best Software & Online Tools — Tested and Reviewed For You. https://bestsoftwaretests.com/how-to-choose-the-best-pilates-app/

How to use pilates stretches to increase your flexibility. (n.d.). Verywell Fit. https://www.verywellfit.com/pilates-stretches-2704728

Is pilates good exercise for osteoarthritis? (n.d.). Verywell Health. https://www.verywellhealth.com/pilates-and-osteoarthritis-2552158

Maddy. (2023, April 21). *3 pilates exercises to help seniors improve balance & mobility - afpa.*

REFERENCES

AFPA. https://www.afpafitness.com/blog/pilates-exercises-help-seniors-improve-balance-mobility/

Nagai, M. (2021, April 28). *Building a pandemic-pilates community - 360 pilates.* 360 Pilates. https://360pilates.com/blog/building-a-pandemic-pilates-community/

Pilates equipment choices for seniors: Safety and effectiveness. (2023, November 6). Pilates Moves You. https://pilatesmovesyou.com/pilates-equipment-choices-for-seniors-safety-and-effectiveness/

Pilates for osteoporosis: Benefits, safety, and risks. (n.d.). Healthline. https://www.healthline.com/health/fitness/pilates-for-osteoporosis

Seven low-impact exercises for seniors. (n.d.). https://www.ourparents.com/senior-health/yoga-and-low-impact-exercise-for-seniors

Soong, K. (2023, January 2). *6 simple steps to build an exercise habit.* Washington Post. https://www.washingtonpost.com/wellness/2023/01/02/exercise-habit-fitness-goals/

Studio reformer konnector - balanced body pilates reformer. (n.d.). https://www.pilates.com/products/studio-reformer-konnector

The impacts of pilates and yoga on health-promoting behaviors and subjective health status. (2021). *International Journal of Environmental Research and Public Health, 18*(7). https://doi.org/10.3390/ijerph18073802

Printed in Great Britain
by Amazon